What About My Weight?

ALSO BY JAMES K. RONE, M.D.

The Thyroid Paradox: How to Get the Best Care for Hypothyroidism

WHAT ABOUT MY WEIGHT?

An Endocrinologist's Unorthodox, Irreverent, Politically Incorrect, Practical Guide to Losing Weight and Combating Obesity

James K. Rone, MD, FACP, FACE
A Member of
The Obesity Society

Arno Press
College Grove, Tennessee

The information contained in this book is based upon the research and personal and professional experiences of the author. It is not intended as a substitute for consulting with your physician or other healthcare provider. Any attempt to diagnose and treat an illness should be done under the direction of a healthcare professional.

The publisher and author do not advocate the use of any particular healthcare protocol to the absolute exclusion of any other but believe the information in this book should be available to the public. The publisher and author are not responsible for any adverse effects or consequences resulting from the use of suggestions, preparations, or procedures discussed in this book. Should the reader have any questions concerning the appropriateness of any procedures or preparation mentioned, the author and publisher strongly suggest consulting a professional healthcare advisor

Arno Press, College Grove, TN 37046
Copyright © 2013 by James K. Rone
All rights reserved. Published 2013

ISBN: 0615892442
ISBN-13: 978-0615892443

For Bill and Bee-Bee…
And my patients.

We have met the enemy and he is us.

—Pogo

CONTENTS

What About My Weight?

INTRODUCTION

My patient might have a thyroid problem, or a cholesterol problem, or I might be seeing him or her for diabetes—we could be dealing with all three—but, regardless, there is an excellent chance the office visit will not end without me being asked this book's title question: "What about my weight, Doc?" or something substantially similar. Until recently, my answer likely as not would have been something pretty short and simple, not too imaginative, especially if the question came as is often the case, at the end of the visit, when I am perhaps late seeing my next patient. I might've replied, for example: "You must take in fewer calories than you burn off."

Which, to be clear, is true advice; it is just not very helpful advice.

Nor is it news to most people. Most people know that particular kernel of wisdom, yet may start to question it, or conclude there is something wrong with them, some disease needing treatment, when they encounter frustrating difficulty, or even out-and-out failure, in their weight-management efforts. I have been a practicing clinical endocrinologist for nearly a quarter century, and it is my observation—especially in recent years, as the epidemic of obesity has gripped the United States, and indeed much of the world, ever more tighteningly—that many, perhaps most of my patients struggle with weight, and not uncommonly become frustrated, sometimes angered, by a perceived lack of success relative to the effort they're putting in.

It has therefore become my mission, and part of the impetus for writing this book, to educate my patients that they *aren't special.* Yes, you read that right, and please don't take it wrongly: every person is of course unique in a vast many ways, and as this book makes clear, every case of obesity is unique, but in the general sense, the person finding their weight management to be a tough road is not a special case. The woman who can't lose weight as seemingly easily as her husband or coworker is not sick. She does not need me to diagnose and treat a disease for her. It is quite rare, in fact, for a medical disorder to be the sole cause of one's obesity, and rarer still to find a disorder that is readily treatable—with say a prescription or surgery—where that therapy is followed, close on its heels, by easy weight loss.

Rather, the woman in the above situation needs to work harder, or at least differently, on her weight problem, than her husband or coworker. 'Tis true, this isn't fair, but it is equally true that fairness is not a relevant concept in the biological sciences. In fact, much in life is not fair. Robert Browning wrote in 1855: "The common problem...everyone's, is—not to fancy what were fair in life provided it could be—but finding first what may be, then find out how to make it fair up to our means."

This book is my answer at last—my good answer, that is—to the title's question *what about my weight?* It is not a short and simple answer like, *you must take in fewer calories than you burn off,* which, as I said, is true as far as it goes. Many factors, however, contributing to the epidemic of obesity are beyond, or largely beyond any one individual's control. A key emphasis of the Blackburn Course in Obesity Medicine, put on annually by Harvard Medical School, is that human energy balance (a fancy term for weight management) is *complex and regulated.* That is, there is involuntary physiology that cannot be voluntarily or readily cast aside by patients in their efforts to control a weight problem. Further complicating weight-loss success, in my view, is a whole raft of misleading information, and pure myth, being promulgated, mucking up the works.

This book details those mitigating factors—mitigating with respect to the commonplace picture of obesity as a simple condition, all or mostly the patient's fault, representative even of a character flaw—and offers suggestions for lessening the impact of such factors. The book's target audience is anybody who is obese or just overweight and struggling to take off the excess. I also include among those who should read and heed this book, anybody whose weight is normal or near normal, but desiring tips on healthier living with the goal of preventing future obesity and obesity-related diseases, and those with loved ones fitting any aforementioned category. And speaking of obesity-related diseases, many overweight and obese patients also suffer from diabetes and/or hyperlipidemia (high cholesterol or triglycerides), to cite just the two my practice would most commonly deal with.

Let me be clear: this is a book about weight, about losing it, and keeping it off.

Period.

It is not a guide for diabetes management nor for lowering your cholesterol.

Be that as it may, a critical part, probably a sine qua non, of effective therapy of those conditions is weight loss, and therefore, many patients with diabetes or hyperlipidemia would benefit from reading *What About My Weight?* And since, being an endocrinologist, many of my patients are diabetic or hyperlipidemic, and since this book is intended to help my patients first and foremost—and those like them for whom I haven't had the honor of treating—there will be points in the text where issues specifically related to obesity management in the diabetic, for example, will be discussed. I will endeavor to keep those comments brief so not to detract from the general-obesity thrust of the book, but in cases where the topic demands more thorough coverage, I will label those clearly, giving the non-diabetic reader the option of skipping ahead.

That said, the vast majority of information herein is equally relevant to the diabetic, the otherwise-ill obese, the healthy overweight or obese, and the normal-proportioned person wanting to learn more about healthy living. In fact, I've often heard it said, a diabetic diet is a healthy diet for everybody. I'll extend that to encompass lifestyle in general; there is little difference in what constitutes healthy living, regardless of whether or not one has been diagnosed with diabetes.

Also a target reader for this book is anyone worried about developing diabetes, or heart disease or stroke, because of a family history of those conditions, or possibly some borderline blood sugars or cholesterols his or her doctor has warned about.

In short, there are few people alive in the United States today who could not benefit from reading *What About My Weight?*

This is a practical book, a bit irreverent with respect to mainstream medical dogma about, for example, fat and alcohol consumption. It is a commonsense approach to weight management, at least my MD version of common sense, and yet it incorporates some of the most cutting edge obesity information coming out of medical research centers in 2013.

Weight-loss books, programs, and schemes, it seems to me, can be divided into two groups: (1) *mainstream*, which won't stray far from a bare-bones, eat-right-and-exercise message, that losing weight involves little more than burning off more calories than one takes in; and (2) *alternative*, wherein all manner of sometimes bizarre tricks, dietary modifications, or supplements are employed to aid weight loss. And, to risk generalizing, I propose that the more reasonable, perhaps more successful of the alternative programs rest on a common theme of "fooling" one's appetite to make it easier to achieve energy balance—a beneficial balance, that is, of calories-in versus calories-out.

Often a particular program's "gimmick" (eliminate carbs, or eliminate fats, or eat grapefruit, or take a magic pill) is presented in isolation, as if that were all one had to do. Yet it is fallacy to believe any single intervention will solve a problem as complex as obesity. Another fallacy is the notion that any given scheme will be universally applicable. There are different solutions for different people. (The Atkinses and Ornishes of the world though would not sell as many books if they plastered a banner across their covers saying: "The perfect diet for *some*!")

The trick to successful weight management is to achieve proper energy balance, and most people don't, nor is it as easy to do so as most patients and, truthfully, most doctors believe it to be. It may even be true that many people *can't* achieve this balance by themselves. I believe we doctors need to do more than just say "eat right and exercise." We need to help our patients balance energy-in and energy-out by showing *why* it's so difficult, introducing some of those appetite-fooling tricks, and helping them seek an effective plan personalized for their genetic background and other individual factors (mainstreamists are as bad as alternativists about preaching "universal" advice).

Above all, we need to manage *expectations*: few, for example, will lose as much weight with diet and exercise as with bariatric surgery—and certainly nobody should be getting frustrated by any failure to do so. Another expectation to be quashed: what worked for one person will work for another. There is in fact an excellent chance it won't.

What About My Weight? does not attempt to present a single unified plan for weight loss. I believe such an approach would be, for most people, doomed to failure. Rather its purpose is to broadly educate on the many and diverse causes of and solutions for obesity, including environmental and food-industry exposures, including ironically, those exposures meant to be helpful, and yet might be the reverse—like sugar-free beverages. Its approach is basically mainstream. To lose weight it is necessary to burn more calories than are consumed. I will beat that drum as hard as anybody, while also covering those mitigating factors that complicate weight management, and can be exploited if properly understood to develop strategies that promote success. In other words, this book acknowledges a business-as-usual, yet only-rarely-successful approach, while augmenting it with a variety of practical, less staid tips, information, and principles.

Above all—I hope it helps and inspires.

1

ENERGY BALANCE

Americans are in deplorable shape and it's everybody's fault.
The public.
Doctors.
Big business.
Big government.

As a board-certified endocrinologist, I have a ringside seat for America's obesity epidemic. Not just America's: "Obesity has emerged as one of the greatest global health challenges of the 21st century," opened a 2012 *New England Journal of Medicine* editorial. Obesity is more prevalent in the countries of the former Soviet Union, and in the Middle East, than the United States. Unhealthy body weight is so common, I don't think we readily recognize it as abnormal anymore—and statistically, perhaps it isn't, but physiologically it is definitely abnormal. It causes more than sixty separate medical disorders, according to Dr. Lee Kaplan, who directs the Massachusetts General Hospital Weight Center. It is a fatal disease. Really notice those around you, and you'll see an astonishing number carrying around excess adiposity (fat tissue), sometimes with difficulty: fatigue, shortness of breath, orthopedic problems. There is a full range of obesity complications: metabolic, structural, inflammatory, arthritic, cancerous, and psychological. And to say obesity is a fatal disease is neither exaggeration nor hype. There has emerged recently the notion of the "metabolically healthy but obese" person; however, at least three papers published in 2013, one in *Diabetes Care*, one in *Obesity*, the last in the *Journal of Clinical Endocrinology and Metabolism*, suggest that these individuals, rather than having a free pass, are only enjoying a temporary reprieve. It is, as states the title of one of those papers, "a matter of time," the data showing that they too are at increased risk of diabetes, and cardiovascular death.

Yet obesity is within our power to control—not easily, don't misunderstand, and perhaps not without help, but within our power nonetheless. That's good news! We just need to figure a way, together, to make it happen. And with few exceptions—individuals whose identities, senses of self-worth, perhaps, are thoroughly wrapped up in being a "big guy" or "big lady," and don't desire a change—most overweight and obese persons, in my experience, are perfectly aware of the problem, and are motivated to change. Nor is it rare to find people fretting about, perhaps inappropriately, body weights within the normal range, owing to a recent, but medically acceptable degree of weight gain, or because they suffer a distorted body image, driven to seek excessive thinness.

In other words, there is widespread awareness and concern, excessively so in some instances, yet weight control—*energy balance*—eludes most obese patients. There are multiple and complex reasons, some *physiological* (that is, normal) and some *pathological* (disease-related). I believe, however, except rarely, everyone is capable of controlling their weight. And if they have tried and failed, if they are disheartened, there is nevertheless nothing mysterious at work. It is simply a reflection of difficult things being difficult, complex things being complicated, slow things being frustrating, and a spate of conflicting expert opinions and erroneous assumptions that confuse and confound the best and brightest of us.

That said, I will relate what was to me, a glaring vignette:

I was awaiting takeoff aboard an airliner. Across the aisle sat a man traveling alone. Fortyish, dressed like a businessman, morbidly obese, squeezed, it seemed to me, uncomfortably in his seat—eating a huge, ingredients-dripping-out, submarine sandwich, with a sizeable bag of chips, and drinking a soda. I know nothing of this man or his health—but, it is hard to imagine him having no health problem(s) related to obesity, including a likely elevated risk of heart attack, stroke, cancer, and diabetes. It is also hard to imagine his physician not advising weight loss. As for his personal goals, I can say nothing, but—again, hard to imagine him not desiring at least some weight reduction.

Yet, as I observed him, his calorie intake seemed to me utterly and obviously excessive, and from a medical standpoint, irresponsible. If I sound insensitive, mocking even, that is not my intent. I am presenting an objective clinical observation out of our current societal milieu. To shy away from such considerations would be a failure to acknowledge all the contributors to, and potential solutions for, what we have already acknowledged to be a global health crisis.

Now, maybe this scenario was unusual for him; maybe this gentleman overeats only when nervously waiting for planes to takeoff, but I doubt it. Weren't there smaller sandwiches in the terminal, and if he really liked *that* one, and really wanted it all, *why add chips?* My point: this man, consciously or not, was his own worst enemy, it seems to me.

I believe, at some level, many who struggle with weight are, as well, their own worst enemies, though they may be completely and honestly unaware of it. I'm not saying all or most of my patients asking advice on weight reduction are overeating to the degree I believe the man on the plane to have been.

But many *are* overeating.

Even if only subtly.

Even if they bitterly deny it.

Now—there are other factors. And we will dig into them. And these other factors make it so that correcting the overeating alone many not cure the obesity. Cutting calories, specifically, and eating healthier, in general, may not alone lead to a healthy weight.

But it is a start, and a necessary one.

HOW MANY CALORIES?

I'm an endocrinologist—an internist subspecialized in diseases of hormones and metabolism. Largely, I deal with thyroid problems and diabetes mellitus, which are areas of medicine most people recognize as ones in which body weight is of concern, either as a cause of, or consequence of the disease.

Thus, I frequently end up talking to patients about weight, whether it be me recommending a reduction, or the patient asking advice. That said, *I do not run a weight-loss clinic.* (Actually, full disclosure, for a brief while recently, I did! My role, though, was temporary and largely administrative.) The point being, weight issues are not the primary focus of the majority of my patient-care interactions. I am not a dietitian, nor any sort of nutritional scientist. If you ask a staffer of a weight-loss clinic, or a dietitian how many calories to consume daily to achieve or maintain a healthy weight, you would no doubt get a specific, numerical, scientifically and arithmetically derived answer that might serve you well. And if pressed, I or my nurse can plug some numbers into a formula and, *voilà*, give you a number as well.

But we almost never do.

Instead, my response when asked *how many calories?* is:

The proof is in the pudding.

Whatever calorie intake results in the desired outcome.

Whatever diet works.

I intend those replies to be neither flippant nor dismissive. In fact, an answer based upon adjusting efforts in light of objective outcomes, is a more likely route to success than any strategy based upon clinging to some calculated number that might or might not have accurately anticipated all the major variables affecting an individual's weight at any given time. Further, I argue that healthcare providers—physician and nonphysician alike, alternativist and mainstreamist—demonstrate much hubris in their pontificating about and advising upon, what I will call, *personal nutritional responsibility*.

Weight management is nothing more and nothing less than manipulating human physiology, which is immensely complex and diverse. Surely if we, the healthcare community, were better at giving nutritional and other lifestyle advice, we'd be achieving better results than we have been combating the epidemic of obesity and related diseases, such as type 2 diabetes. I for one would prefer less dogmatism, less posturing, fewer complicated, sometimes expensive schemes, and a lot more common sense—on everyone's part, patient and provider alike.

THE SCIENCE OF EVERYTHING

Physics is the science of everything—the basis of all science, including biology and medicine. Two physics principles relevant to human body weight are: (1) *the law of conservation of mass-energy*, and (2) *the second law of thermodynamics*. The first is a fundamental inescapable truism. The second, while not negating the first, explains how we, in a manner of speaking, get to cheat the first. See Appendix A for a more comprehensive discussion of these physics laws and their relevance in obesity. For the purposes of this chapter I will be brief.

Not to put too fine a point on it: the first of these principles tell us that matter, that is, body weight, is neither created nor destroyed. The second says that the imposed, energy-maintained orderliness, which is one of the features that distinguishes life from non-life in our universe, makes it so that we can easily and readily increase our mass, or body weight.

I didn't say, *create* body weight.

I said, *increase* body weight.

A huge difference.

Our bodies put on weight for all kinds of reasons, from all kinds of sources, but there is not an ounce of weight gain, ever, that is not the result of intake: something having been swallowed. Matter is neither created nor destroyed. (Again, see Appendix A, or else you'll just have to trust me on that one.)

Now, the only weight gain this book is really concerned with is fat weight.

Adiposity.

Adipose tissue being a fancy term for fat.

People can gain weight from building muscle. That doesn't bother me. That is not obesity. People can gain water weight, from water they have swallowed, especially if they also swallowed salt. Salt tends to help us retain water. Water is matter and has weight, but it has no calories. Water weight, which can be a medical problem, is not the medical problem this book deals with. This book deals with obesity—excess adiposity. This is fundamentally important. Excess body weight, or a high *body mass index*, a term we'll define later, is not the same thing as *obesity*.

Obesity is an excess of body fat that predisposes to obesity-related disease. Body weight and body mass index are measurements, not diseases. They are determined by fat in the body, but also, by the weight of bone, and muscle, and internal organs, and the brain, and body water. If a person weighs more than average simply because she has an exceptionally thick bone structure, or better built muscles, or because she is retaining excess water and salt, that person is not obese. That person is not at increased risk of, for instance, diabetes. A person's legs ballooning up with fluid retention, edema, is a medical problem, but not obesity, not a problem to be dealt with in this book, nor by an endocrinologist, generally, nor an obesity-medicine specialist.

I make this point because I have had patients get angry at me for not addressing their increased weight that was clearly due to water retention, not fatty excess, nothing putting them at risk of obesity-related disease. These patients might need to see their internist, might need a diuretic to get off some fluid, but that is not an obesity-medicine or obesity-treatment issue. These folks are making body weight and obesity equivalent, when they are not. All obesity is associated with excess body weight, but not all excess body weight is obesity.

The only weight that matters to the obesity specialist, the only weight that matters here, is fat weight. The first rule of medical therapy is knowing what we are treating. Without that, we are far less likely to reach a satisfying outcome.

The Conservation Law

A *calorie*, in the manner we will, and most laypeople use the term, is the quantity of energy required to raise one kilogram of water (about a quart) by one Celsius degree. A calorie is, therefore, a unit of energy. As we go forward, I will use the terms *calorie* and *energy* largely interchangeably. Thus, if I say, "to lose weight one must decrease energy intake and increase energy expenditure," that is the same thing as saying, "…one must decrease calorie intake and increase calorie expenditure," and that is the same thing as saying, "…one must eat less and exercise more."

In nutritional terms, energy is both good and bad. We must have energy; that is, we must take in calories. Without energy we can't work, think, move, play, heal wounds, generate body heat; in short, we can't sustain or live life. But if we take in too much energy, and fail to burn it off somehow, we store it as fat, possibly overwhelming our fat-storing mechanisms, causing a fatty infiltration of internal organs, such as the liver and pancreas, even muscles, leading to widespread illness and dysfunction. *Energy balance*, which I've already defined very loosely as *weight control*, is defined by physiologists as the relation of the amount of usable energy taken into the body to that employed for internal work, external work, and the growth and repair of tissues. *Negative energy balance*, where intake minus output (that is, swallowed calories minus calories burned doing work, or other functions) is a negative number, results in weight loss—a loss of the total amount of energy in the body. *Positive energy balance*, where intake exceeds output, results in weight gain. The ideal situation, assuming one is currently at a healthy weight, is *zero energy balance*, neither weight gain nor weight loss, calories-in equaling calories-out. Weight control.

So, understanding energy, the body's obtaining of it, channeling of it, storing of it, is key to understanding obesity, and its prevention and treatment. If you've been paying close attention up to now, you may have been struck by a confusing point: *why am I talking about energy, when what you and I and this book are concerned with is weight?* Weight meaning mass, or matter, or stuff—stuff you can take in your hands, feel the texture of, the heft of. Can you feel energy? Well, you can feel kinetic energy when a hammer smashes your thumbnail. You can feel thermal energy when your hand gets too close to a hot stove. But you can't weigh energy, and this book is concerned with nothing if not, primarily, stuff you can weigh.

When I say you can't weigh energy, that statement is true within everyday experience, and that's fine for our purposes. This book does not deal with issues outside everyday experience. Now, to a nuclear physicist or theoretical physicist, energy actually does have mass—it can be weighed—and mass has energy. The two are interchangeable (see Appendix A). Our bodies however, don't get to tap into that energy; only nuclear reactors, and atom bombs, and stars, like our sun, get to convert significant amounts of matter wholesale into energy.

When I talk about calories and energy and body weight, I'm talking about, for example, a certain number of grams of some foodstuff, which is *eaten*, and increases one's body weight by that number of grams. The body then *digests* that foodstuff, so it can *absorb* the usable nutrients into the bloodstream, which transports them to some cell, say a left quadriceps muscle cell. Those usable nutrients probably weigh something less than the original number of grams of the foodstuff, some of that mass having remained behind in the intestines as fiber.

Those usable nutrients, in that quadriceps muscle, are then *metabolized*. There are numerous possible metabolic fates, but let's assume for this simple illustration there is an immediate need for energy to do muscle work—at that very moment the person is doing leg presses at the gym. The nutrients are metabolized to energy. When that happens, some of the chemical bonds that hold together the atoms making up the nutrient molecules, are broken, and release energy. That energy is captured by the body in the formation of new chemical compounds, such as *adenosine triphosphate*, or ATP, the body's main energy currency. The total amount of energy releasable, either immediately or eventually, by those usable nutrients, is expressed as the number of calories contained in the number of grams of the original foodstuff.

Up to this point no mass has been lost by the body.

The grams of foodstuff have become an equal total number of

grams of colonic fiber plus usable nutrients and now those nutrients have been split into smaller molecules, whose mass sums to the same total as the original usable nutrients. Energy, chemical energy, has been released, but that does not change mass. This biochemical energy comes from *splitting molecules*—that is, *splitting bonds between atoms*, not *splitting atoms*. When atoms are split (fission) or slammed together (fusion) to form new atoms, that's when mass is lost, and flitters off into massive amounts of energy, the stuff that happens in nuclear reactors and the center of the sun. In our bodies, though, the chemical energy released in metabolic processes is small potatoes. No measureable amount of mass is directly lost.

The end products of general energy metabolism, however, include carbon dioxide and water. Carbon dioxide and water are both breathed out via the lungs and water of course leaves the body in all sorts of ways, including substantially in the form of sweat and urine.

So, when nutrients are metabolized to meet energy needs, the original ingested mass of the foodstuff leaves the body in the form of (1) fecal matter, (2) exhaled carbon dioxide, and (3) water-containing fluids. No weight is gained. Zero energy balance.

Say as a result of those leg presses, the quadriceps bulks up. In that case, some of those nutrients are metabolized into new muscle-fiber proteins—positive energy balance (a good version of positive energy balance, by the way). Say, on the other hand, those leg presses were skipped and there was no energy or bulking-up need. Then all or a significant portion of the nutrients might be stored as fat (a bad form, from an obesity-medicine perspective, of positive energy balance). Lastly, say, so many leg-presses were performed that the ingested nutrients couldn't meet the energy demand. In that case, stored glycogen and/or fat would have to be metabolically mobilized to make up the energy deficit. Negative energy balance, and body weight would decline.

At no point in all of this was any matter or energy created or destroyed. Right? A bunch of molecules were swallowed, digested, and metabolized, to a bunch of different molecules, with some energy released along the way. Energy that was there in the foodstuff, as potential energy, to begin with. Nothing created nor destroyed.

That is the *conservation law.*

A fundamental law of the universe.

And it is critical for the purposes of this book that you understand and embrace that law. It means any weight gained by a human being was either food eaten, or water drunk. Period. People don't gain weight out of thin air. Some organisms "fix" nitrogen out of the air—humans can't. We absorb oxygen through our lungs, but for every oxygen molecule inhaled, we exhale one carbon dioxide—a heavier molecule.* If anything, then, breathing is a weight losing proposition. Besides the oxygen/carbon-dioxide exchange, the muscles of respiration burn calories, and even in terms of water weight, breathing is a route of fluid loss.

I make this point so strongly and longwindedly because it is truly common, nearly daily, that a patient complains to me in distress that she has gained *x* number of pounds "without eating a thing," or pleads, "I'm eating *right*" or "*healthy*" or "*the way I should.*"

Drop the Hyperbole!

With all due respect...

Don't take yourself out of the loop.

There may be some reason why it is harder for you to lose weight than somebody else, but there is no human disease, nor physiological variegation, that creates weight out of thin air—mass is neither created nor destroyed—if you gained it, you swallowed it. Don't try to convince me or anybody else, least of all yourself, that you didn't. You cannot solve a problem you don't acknowledge all the major contributors to.

Everybody eats and drinks.

Many of us do it to excess.

Even if not to obvious excess, everybody still eats and drinks (except terminal cancer and AIDS patients, and the wretchedly poor, none of whom are subjects of this book). If you gained weight, you ate more than you burned off, or you drank more water than you urinated, sweated, or breathed out, or both.

You might be eating "right" by most people's estimation, but that doesn't matter, and you must stop thinking it does. And that's where my proof-is-in-the-pudding, outcome-based approach has advantages. It gets away from what "should be" into "what is." If you aren't losing weight, don't focus on what "should work," focus on changing whatever it is you are doing, until you find something

---

* Not entirely true, but enough so. For the record, a variable amount of inhaled oxygen is converted to carbon dioxide, the average being 82 percent (a value known as the *respiratory quotient*)—the rest is converted to water, which exits via lungs, skin, and kidneys.

that does work.

So, the conservation law does apply. Body weight never forms out of thin air. Consumption of calories, energy intake, is necessary to see an increase in body weight, especially an increase in fat weight. Does, however, harping and focusing incessantly and exclusively upon that consumption necessarily improve an unhealthy weight?

No. To the contrary, the conservation law, while it does apply, is buried under layer upon layer of complex human physiology, confusing things, mucking up the works. Many factors, including a labyrinth of appetite regulating and reward signals, and varying degrees of insulin resistance, to name only two such factors, machinate behind the scenes to increase energy intake or reduce energy expenditure, often challenging our best efforts and intentions.

The usual approach to weight management is to preach diet and exercise. In extreme cases historically unsafe drugs might be prescribed to cut appetite and intake, or a surgical procedure might be performed to accomplish the same. Each of these modalities is typically employed from the point of view that patients aren't doing their part. That it's all calories in and calories out. That a given outcome is ultimately the result of a given energy balance:

Intake minus output. It is, but controlling that outcome, achieving that negative or zero energy balance is much more than that, much more any simple equation.

It is more complicated.

Meaning that a person can be doing their level best to match calories-in with calories-out and still not achieve their desired energy balance. The how and why of that and how to get through that quagmire is the subject of this book.

The Second Law

We've discussed the conversion law, that matter is never created nor destroyed. The other physics law we are concerning ourselves with is the *second law of thermodynamics*—what I will call, *the second law*, and again, see Appendix A for further explanation.

The second law deals with *entropy*.

It specifically says all processes of change in the universe tend toward *increasing entropy*.

Entropy is a degree of disorder, growing with time, irreversibly. And this offers, I think, an elegant explanation for how human obesity can seem so readily to violate the conservation law—not really violate it, but put on a good show of it. How, when matter is neither created nor destroyed, people can still gain weight, despite a conscientious effort not to, without it being entirely their fault.

Entropy is the answer.

Or rather, our lack of it, life being by definition a *low-entropy* proposition.

Biology 101:

University of South Carolina, Dr. Wallace Dawson:

"Life is a *low-entropy* potentially self-replicating homeostatic system maintained by energy flow through it."

Entropy wins in the long run, but we living humans, wedged between birth and death, get to cheat, get to enjoy that powerful overlay of human behavior and physiology and genetics and pathology and technology and economics and culture that buffer us.

The *bio-psycho-sociology of obesity*, if you will, temporarily trumps the *physics of obesity*. The physics is real, and it applies. But our bodies are awfully skilled, conniving even, at manipulating the system—implanting insatiable cravings in our minds, for instance, or furtively reducing resting energy expenditure for the expressed purpose of subverting short-term weight-loss successes—at making end runs around the physics, whether we want that or not.

In short, *our bodies are awfully good at gaining weight*.

SCIENCE AND ART

I am a clinical physician. All my professional time is spent seeing patients, and it is from this perspective of seeing patients day in and day out that this book was born—a book presenting my observations, speculations, experiences, pet peeves, tips and techniques, and some science, related to weight management, gleaned from my personal life, and over a quarter century of clinical experience.

It is not my purpose to dogmatically espouse "rules" for controlling weight, or some rigid protocol, or "diet," because to propose uniform directives for every person would apply an inappropriate level of simplicity and uniformity to a complex, nonuniform problem. At the heart of that complexity lies the diversity of biology in general and humanity in particular. People have different shaped noses, eye colors, skin tones, personalities, and they have different causes of and solutions for their weight issues.

One of the big problems I see in effectively managing obesity is an unfortunate hubris regarding our understanding of and ability to control all the relevant factors. I see this in both healthcare providers and patients. It is folly to try to control every calorie to the nth degree, or define any one best nutritional plan. There is a popular book out there about eating differently depending on one's blood type. I don't say I agree with all it says, but the notion that a person's best nutritional plan varies with genetic factors is entirely simpatico with my criticism of our typical too-simple, too-uniform approaches to weight.

I will not present herein a rigorous scientific treatise. I will make no attempt to provide a comprehensive "evidence-based" foundation for the information provided. Don't misunderstand—I must and will cite experts' statements, and the results and conclusions of published scientific papers, to support my points. You should expect that of me and any author claiming scientific expertise, and you should take with a grain of salt any pontificating made without reasonable circumspection, and supportive referencing. Be that as it may, what is presented in *What About My Weight?* is a mix of observations, informed opinions, and evidence— the latter when and where it exists. *Evidence-based medicine* is much touted these days. It seeks peer-reviewed scientific data to support what we do to and for our patients. That's an exceedingly nice idea; however, we don't have rigorous data to cover all situations. To suppose that we do demonstrates, again, extraordinary hubris, and I might argue we don't have it for most situations, if you parse out the details. Oversimplifying complexity yet again.

That said, my discussions are grounded in, and will not deliberately contradict any of my medical-school, residency, and fellowship training, nor decades of continuing medical education. There is no hocus-pocus here—yet, *medicine is both science and art.*

Even in the 21st century. Good medicine is both science and art.

Bad medicine excludes either in favor of the other.

There is science to managing one's weight, and there is art.

This book deals with both, and it may not be obvious which is which.

2

THE BIOLOGY OF OBESITY

Before we dive into how to prevent or correct obesity, let's step back and briefly overview what we're up against. Most of us—myself included, until very recently—harbor a very simple, traditional view of human energy balance and weight management. That traditional view is that it's all about *energy intake* versus *energy expenditure*. Energy intake is everything we swallow that has calories; energy expenditure is all calories burned, whether at rest or during voluntary work or exercise.

That view is highly incomplete. Human body weight is not simple; it is, in the words of Harvard's Dr. Lee Kaplan, "complex and regulated." That *regulated* part, is especially important. It means our bodies actively regulate our weight, try to keep it stable, largely behind the scenes, subconsciously—just as our bodies, when healthy, regulate our serum sodium level within a narrow normal range without us giving it a thought, or our internal body temperature. It is not even true that the person whose weight is rock stable is taking in exactly the number of calories needed, day in and day out, to run their physiology and physical activities. *How likely does that seem, in fact?* Human adults, and all adult mammals, it turns out, routinely eat as many as three times more calories than are needed. That excess is necessary as a reserve, in case, say a bear chases you through the woods. This means the person eating a 2500-calorie diet is burning off an excess of around 1700 calories every day, the equivalent of seventeen miles of running.

A complicated network of signals traveling between the gut and the brain and fat tissue and even muscle accomplishes this regulation, establishing energy balance around a *set point*. That set point, programmed into the hypothalamus of the brain, is defended, and defended well, whether or not the set-point weight is a healthy weight.

By that I mean, if you are obese and weigh around 300 pounds pretty consistently, then your set point is around 300 pounds. If you overeat at the holidays and gain to 310, all those signals are going to start zipping around and work to bring you back to your set point of 300 pounds. If you diet and exercise and lose down to 290, same thing in reverse, those signals increase appetite and decrease basal metabolism, until the weight goes back to the set point. In short, weight gain will almost always decrease regulated energy intake and increase regulated energy expenditure until the set-point weight is again reached, at which point calories in and calories out are once again equal. That's a good thing. The flip side, the bad part, the frustrating part, is that weight loss to below the set point, will almost always increase energy intake and decrease energy expenditure, subconsciously, until the weight is regained. A phenomenon many of my patients can attest to having experienced.

The only obesity treatments that work over the long-term, are those managing to alter the set point. It isn't enough to cut calories and exercise—the brain literally needs to be reprogrammed. Figuring out just how to do that it still a work in progress for all of us.

SIGNALS AND SITES OF REGULATION

As mentioned, a network of hormonal and neuronal signals operate between several organ systems to regulate human body weight. In addition, there are a number of external factors which impact the system: emotions, medications that promote weight gain, food characteristics and availability, habits and behaviors, and environmental cues, including advertising.

I want to spend the remainder of this chapter giving you a sense of the major signals and regulators of energy intake and expenditure, and where they operate.

The Gut

It seems reasonable to start with the gastrointestinal tract (GI tract), which—other than the smell and taste receptors in the nose and mouth, which are involved in all this as well—is the first major contact between the body and food. Fascinatingly, one of the early components of the GI tract to interact with our diet is the so-called *gut microbiota*, the bacteria that inhabit our large and small intestines. There are ten times more bacterial cells, microbes, in and on a human body than human cells, carrying 150 times more genetic information that the entire human genome. And it has recently been appreciated that microbes in the gut function as an organ in and of themselves, exerting important influences on energy balance and fat deposition. They are involved in detoxification of carcinogens, facilitating nutrient absorption, and metabolizing vitamins, drugs, and some internally produced hormones. In short, the gut microbiota may be a major player in human disease and longevity.

It should come as no surprise that one of the functions of the gut microbiota is to help metabolize our diet. It literally burns off some of our ingested calories before they even reach our bloodstreams; the proverbial increase in intestinal gas resulting from eating beans is, for example, the result of gas-producing bacteria helping to digest that foodstuff. Changes in the microbiota and its interaction with bile, a digestive juice released from the liver and gall bladder in response to a fatty meal, seem to affect the tendency toward obesity. We will revisit the gut microbiota in Chapter 9.

Other GI-tract factors operating on weight regulation include stretch receptors in the stomach and duodenum, which signal the brain via the vagus nerve, and reduce appetite. A number of gut hormones are released in response to food, suppressing further intake. These include: *cholecystokinin* from the duodenum, *peptide YY* from the lower small bowel and colon, and *glucagon-like peptide-1* (GLP1) from the small bowel. A rise in *insulin* inhibits appetite but the resulting fall in glucose later in the wake of a meal stimulates it. *Ghrelin* is released by the stomach in the fasted state, peaking just before a meal, helping to produce what we know as hunger. Ghrelin is an appetite-stimulating, or *orexigenic* factor.

Adipose Tissue

Not immediately upon eating, but as fat stores increase, *adipocytes* (fat cells) release the hormone *leptin*, which travels to the hypothalamus of the brain, triggering a number of events, including reduction of certain appetite-stimulating signals, and release of appetite reducers and metabolism stimulators, the latter including thyroid-hormone regulators and the sympathetic neurotransmitter, norepinephrine.

Central Signals

When an endocrinologist says *central*, he or she often means the brain, more specifically the hypothalamus. Below is a list of centrally released appetite signals segregated according to the direction of their effect. I present this list not with the intent that you memorize it, or even attempt to understand how these things do what they do. It is enough that you appreciate how complex body-weight regulation is.

- Substances that stimulate feeding
  - Neuropeptide Y
  - Agouti-related protein
- Substances that decrease feeding
  - Melanocyte-stimulating hormone
  - Serotonin
  - Norepinephrine
  - Corticotropin-releasing hormone
  - Cocaine- and amphetamine-regulated transcript

The Adrenal Glands

The major adrenal steroid *cortisol* is released in response to eating and is a stimulator of further feeding. Cortisol excess is a well-known promoter of obesity.

Skeletal Muscle

I'll bet, like me, you never thought of skeletal muscle as an endocrine organ. It turns out that even muscle generates a substance, a hormone, that regulates body weight. Muscle in fact talks to fat. Muscle when subjected to exercise releases a hormone called *irisin*, which causes the conversion of ordinary "white" fat to a "brown-fat-like" tissue that burns more calories through body-heat production.

Obesity is Heterogeneous

Hopefully this brief chapter has demonstrated the complexity and distribution body-wide of the responses to and the modulators of body weight, and metabolism, and energy balance. I encourage you to look back on this information when considering whether any one intervention is likely to be a solution to your weight issues. Thyroid hormone, for example. I treat many patients for hypothyroidism, including those whose findings are rather subtle or cryptic. Sometimes I hope to, and sometimes I succeed in, affecting body weight in my thyroid-treated patients. However, there are many other factors, and it is clear that the mechanisms of and solutions for obesity vary widely from individual to individual. For weight management to succeed it is critical to recognize that what works for one, likely will *not* work for the next. It is critical to be open-minded and flexible, and primed to try the next different thing or combination of things as soon as the last is shown to have failed.

3

"BUDGET" YOUR CALORIES

An analogy can be drawn between personal weight management and personal financial management. Both disciplines deal with bits of something valuable going in and out, with the goal of balancing inflow and outflow in some beneficial way. One, interestingly, mirror-images the other—the biggest challenges lying on opposite sides of the in/out equation.

In personal finance, we try to maximize income, of course, but that side of the equation is often fixed, or at least difficult to change, and not always in the individual's immediate power to change. The common challenge is on the outflow side—overspending being very easy, and often pleasurable, and budget-balancing being largely dependent upon curbing such urges.

In weight management, it is the energy-expenditure side, calorie-burning, or "spending" side that is largely fixed. More calories can be burned by increasing exercise, but a real impact is difficult to achieve. It is the energy-intake side, the consuming of calories that must be limited, in opposition to powerful "pleasure-center"-reinforced drives.

There is a personal-finance guru in my local area named Dave Ramsey. He is a bestselling author and host of a nationally syndicated radio show. I've heard him say on the radio many times that personal finance is 90 percent behavior and 10 percent math (or something like that, I'm paraphrasing). He repeats this whenever a caller comes out of the woodwork with some scheme to get out of debt faster using a lower-interest credit card, or rewards card, or no-interest financing, or whatever.

No matter how airtight the caller's math, Mr. Ramsey's position always is that it is better to just line up the bills, pay them till they're gone, than it is to get bogged down in all that math minutia, saving small amounts here and there on interest.

The math is a distraction at best, a trap at worst.

So too it is with weight management. The habits, the actions, are more important than the math. To accurately track all calories in and out, day in and day out, is a Herculean task. Few people are going to do it well, far fewer for long enough to accomplish a meaningful durable outcome. And anybody who did do all that wouldn't be leaving much focus for the rest of a fulfilling life.

Add to that the physiological likelihood that a sustained reduction in calories will be countered by a reduced energy expenditure by the body, a decreased metabolism, and any lost weight will likely be regained.

I do not believe detailed tracking and recording of calories is a path to success for most people struggling with weight. That said, an important and repeating message of this book is that different things work for different people. If counting calories and recording them to the nth degree works for you, and I mean really, objectively is working, over a sustained period of time—not just wishful-thinking working—great! Do it. But if things aren't falling into place, stop counting and try a different strategy.

A patient recently showed me her calorie-counting smartphone "app" that graphed in extraordinary detail her day-by-day ins and outs, her concern being that she was doing all this and not losing weight. I was able to point out, on her smart phone, that there were many days where she consumed a thousand calories more than her average of 1800 or so. And since it takes about a 500-calorie-per-day deficit to lose one pound per week, each of my patient's thousand-calorie-up days was a two-day backtrack.

Problem explained.

She didn't seem to embrace my point—but, further, it seemed to me she was missing the big picture, buried in all those conscientiously tracked numbers. A strategy that she herself was telling me wasn't working for her.

I think it's usually better to focus on food choice and portion size and being more active and maintaining good habits in general than to get bogged down in numbers, which is why I hardly ever give a patient a calorie-intake prescription.

4

NUTRITIONAL MANAGEMENT DOESN'T MEAN "GO ON A DIET"

Merriam-Webster's Collegiate Dictionary, 11th ed., offers several definitions of the noun *diet*. Three are as follows: (1) food and drink regularly provided or consumed, (2) habitual nourishment, and (3) a regimen of eating and drinking sparingly so as to reduce one's weight. The origin of *diet* is from the Greek *diaita*, meaning "manner of living."

Most people use *diet* according to the third definition, as in, "After the holidays I'm going on a diet to lose twenty pounds," implying something temporary. After the twenty pounds is lost they stop the "diet" and return to their regular habits, regular habits that got them to the point they felt they needed to lose the twenty pounds in the first place. If those habits are restored without any sustained modification, they will regain the twenty pounds.

Diet roller coaster and *yo-yo dieting* are terms applied to this common scenario. Now, if a person lost and regained the same twenty pounds again and again, wobbling persistently between some hypothetical acceptable weight and "acceptable plus twenty," I suppose that person wouldn't be much less healthy than a twin who maintained throughout life an ideal *body mass index* (BMI, a composite of weight and height). Unfortunately, a frequent consequence of the diet roller coaster is a *net increase* in BMI over time, accomplishing nothing in terms of enhancing one's health.

I prefer to think of a diet as something sustained, as in definitions (1) and (2), and consistent with the word's *manner-of-living* etymology. The person vowing to lose twenty pounds, under my paradigm, would not "go on a diet" but would "change diets." Permanently, so the twenty pounds is never regained. It is more difficult to make a permanent change than to do something for a week or month or three months, but it is more likely to be successful in ways that are medically important. "Obesity is best conceptualized as a chronic condition," wrote the authors of a January 2013 paper in the *New England Journal of Medicine*, "requiring ongoing management to maintain long-term weight loss."

MEDICALLY SIGNIFICANT WEIGHT MANAGEMENT

My concern, as a physician, is the short- and long-term health of patients. Thus my involvement in their body-weight management is limited to helping them achieve or maintain an acceptable BMI, an acronym I will often use in place of *weight*, since it is more medically relevant. *Weight* is an absolute number of pounds, which by itself doesn't tell much. Say my patient weighs 150 pounds. If he is a man six-feet-two-inches tall, 150 pounds is low-normal for him. But if she is a five-foot-zero woman, she is borderline obese. Thus, for medical purposes—for identifying and controlling risk factors for obesity-related diseases—we need a simple way of combining a person's weight and height in a meaningful expression.

Hence, BMI—kilograms body weight divided by the square of the person's height in meters ($BMI = kg/m^2$). Nobody calculates this on their own, by the way. The computer in my office calculates it on my patients, and you can easily find a chart to determine yours in any number of books, or on the Internet. An ideal BMI is around 22, while BMIs above 26 or 27 are associated with two- to six-fold increases in risk for hypertension, hypercholesterolemia, and diabetes. A BMI of 30 or greater generally defines obesity, whereas 40 or greater is considered "morbid" obesity, or Class III obesity (Classes I and II being defined by a BMI of 30.0–34.9 and 35.0–39.9, respectively). And obesity-medicine specialists are currently seeing an alarming increase in patients with BMIs greater than 50. There are as many people in the United States with a BMI over 50 (termed *super obesity*) as are diagnosed every year with HIV positivity, or Parkinson's disease.

Any numerical distinctions are somewhat arbitrary—the upper limit of normal for BMI is often defined as 24.9, for instance—but it is safe to say the more the BMI exceeds 26 or 27, the greater that person's risk for hypertension, hypercholesterolemia, and diabetes, and hence their danger of suffering a heart attack, stroke, or premature death. *It is therefore medically important to lower the BMI of anyone registering above 26 or 27.*

By how much?

From a practical standpoint, any reduction is helpful. A loss of total body weight of only 10 to 20 percent, in some cases less, may dramatically lessen the risk of bad outcomes. A woman who is 5'4", with a BMI of 40, would weigh 235 pounds. If she were to lose 15 percent of her body weight, that would get her to 200 pounds, where she would be a lot healthier (i.e., she would have a lot lower chance of suffering a heart attack or dying in the coming few years), but that would still leave her BMI at 34, still well in the obese range.

We might prefer to get her to 145 pounds (BMI 25), but from a starting point of 235 pounds she is more likely to lose 35 pounds to 200, and keep it off (avoiding the diet roller coaster) than she is 90 pounds to 145. I say this fully aware that research has not proven that correcting "unrealistic" goals helps patients have better outcomes, and in fact several studies show that more ambitious goals can result in more weight loss. So, if our hypothetical patient wants to set a personal long-term goal of losing 90 pounds, fine. But the medically important goal is that first 35 pounds because it is more easily achievable and carries the greatest percentage benefit in terms of long-term health.

One study of young women at high risk of diabetes, for instance, showed that a mean body-weight loss of only 7 percent reduced the appearance of diabetes by 60 percent. In terms of our hypothetical woman (5'4", 235 lb, BMI 40) that 7 percent would leave her at 218 pounds, BMI 37. Yet she likely won't get diabetes, thus preserving her eyesight and kidney function, and lowering her risk of amputation, heart attack, stroke and death. That's a lot of bang for the buck.

Small changes in BMI, therefore, may be of more medical importance than large ones.

Personal Goals Versus Therapeutic Goals

If you are a patient in an endocrinology clinic or your friendly internist's office, a weight loss lowering your BMI from, say, 40 to 35 is of medical importance, as would be a change from 32 to 27. On the other hand, a weight-loss goal lowering the BMI from 24 to 22 (for our hypothetical lady that's 140 pounds down to 130), would not be of much medical consequence, and to be blunt, should not be a topic of discussion during an office visit paid for by health insurance in this era of spiraling expenditures and headlines full of healthcare-financing worries.

Don't misunderstand: I don't believe there is anything wrong with our 140-pound lady wanting to lose ten pounds; I have no objections to cosmetic weight loss, provided the goals are safe (not shooting for a low BMI—we call that an eating disorder) and pursued safely (no dangerous diets, or irresponsible drug use). So long as we remember this is cosmetic, not of medical importance, not done for the purpose of staving off heart attack, stroke, and death.

Nor would I fault anyone desiring responsible cosmetic weight loss going to a competently run, MD/DO-operated clinic dedicated to assisting them. That's not what I do in the Endocrinology Clinic, nor is it what this book is devoted to. The difference is analogous to seeing a general surgeon to have your diseased gall bladder removed, versus a plastic surgeon for, say, a purely aesthetic breast augmentation.

Transient Versus Permanent Changes

While it might be okay to alter one's nutritional intake temporarily to achieve a cosmetic weight-loss goal, any serious effort to reduce BMI for disease-risk reduction must be sustained, must include permanent alterations to one's lifestyle. And since human nature dictates that any behavior change intended to be permanent must be more modest and palatable than anything meant to be tolerated for only short periods, it follows that medically important weight loss will be *slow weight loss.*

One pound per week is the usual recommendation. Patience is a virtue, my mother preached. Because these changes are less dramatic, more palatable, they will be more readily sustained, and more readily become habit. Success, after all, breeds adherence. Thus, slow weight loss will less likely be regained. Referring to the challenge of paying off a huge debt, I've heard Dave Ramsey quip:

"How do you eat an elephant? A bite at a time."

How do you get your BMI down, and keep it down?

A pound at a time.

Besides smaller changes being easier to stick with, hopefully taking root as habit, another reason slow BMI reduction is more likely to last, in my opinion, is that any protocol resulting in a rapid fall in weight has to involve some big intervention. Fast voluntary weight loss requires a large calorie reduction—achieved through some strategy, herculean willpower, or pills, or meal replacement "milk shakes," or major shift in macronutrient balance (macronutrients are fats, carbohydrates, and proteins). Examples might be *no carbs*, or *no fats*, or *all sausage* (kidding). No matter how effective, reasonable, scientifically valid any such intervention might be in the short run, it will never be safe or practical over the long. Yet it requires a lot of effort and focus for whatever length of time it is maintained. Worse, perhaps it requires no effort or focus at all—in the case of, say, some powerful metabolism-stimulating pill.

At the end of this rapid weight-loss program let's presume fifty pounds have been lost. The goal is met, program stopped. But since no effort went into learning new healthy habits, only in enforcing the weird unsustainable protocol, the old unhealthy habits automatically kick back in.

The weight will be regained.

There will have been no lasting value to the effort.

Better, I think, to focus on new *sustainable* habits from the get-go, developing and maintaining them, and let the weight loss come in its own good time. Dr. Lee Kaplan of Harvard says we need to be slowing our patients down, not speeding them up. Don't put the cart before the horse. The cart is a lower BMI, the horse is the lifestyle that gets us there.

Keep the horse out front always.

5

IT'S MOSTLY BUT NOT ALL DIET: MORE HEALTHY LIFESTYLE HABITS

There are two sides to energy balance: intake and expenditure. The swallowing of calories on one side of the teeter-totter, the burning of calories on the other. The last chapter dealt with "diet"—the calories-in side—and I advised small, sustained modifications to nutritional lifestyle. These can be accomplished through self-directed efforts, or should those fail, assistance can be sought from a dietitian, a health-coach, or a commercially available program, such as the well-respected Weight Watchers.

We can have an analogous discussion about the calories-out side: by which we mostly mean *exercise*, or what might better be thought of as *physical-activity habits*.

GET PHYSICAL

There will be more to say in the next chapter about exercise and its relative importance compared to nutrition in comprehensive weight management. For now my message is simple: look for ways to be active, rather than the opposite.

Make activity a habit; don't always put it off for some formal exercise session, a visit to the gym, or jog around the neighborhood. Now, I would never discourage any uninjured person—without significant heart disease, that is, or very brittle bones from advanced osteoporosis—from taking on a formal structured-exercise program like running a few times a week, or going to the fitness center, or riding a stationary bike, or swimming, or training for a marathon, whatever—as long as they actually do it, safely, and regularly, and stick with it over the long run.

Like with nutrition:

Slow, and steady, and sustained is best.

For many people, though, it might be more practical to find ways to incorporate small doses of increased activity, as a matter of routine, throughout the day. Experts call this "lifestyle activity." Get into the *habit* of burning more calories whenever and wherever possible.

Suggestions:

Walk. Often. A quick walk around your workplace parking lot at lunchtime. When you do walk, walk briskly. *Never ever* idle in a parking lot, polluting the planet, wasting fossil fuels, waiting for somebody to back out of a spot close to the store—park out and walk, farther the better. Same with drive-thru's. If you must eat at McDonald's, go inside. Convenience is almost always the enemy of health and BMI.

Speaking of convenience...

Avoid like the plague those conveniences we build for skirting exertion, like elevators and escalators. Take the stairs when you can, and if you are on an escalator, walk it (I really don't care what the sign says). If you live in a two-story house, jog upstairs when you go, and don't let items (books, packages, and so forth) sit at the bottom of the staircase; take them up, whether you were going up then or not.

Ride that exercise bike, or walk that treadmill—for thirty minutes when you can, ten if you don't have time for more, or better yet, several ten-minute sessions through the day. Break up prolonged sitting with bouts of light-to-moderate exercise. A walk perhaps, or just standing to do a task instead of sitting. When I have hours of computer work ahead of me in the office, I take a laptop out to the nurse's station counter and stand doing some of it. I keep a bench press and free weights in my study and take a break from my writing desk a few times a day, a few minutes at a time, running through a simple routine.

Bottom line: barring some significant orthopedic problem or other chronic illness that limits activity, never look for ways to avoid exertion. To the contrary, seek it. Combining the above is best—a formal training regimen mixed with lighter simpler activities, but never take a whole day off from trying to be active.

GET REST TOO

When it comes to lifestyle impacting energy balance, nutrition and physical activity are obviously important categories. A less obvious, less discussed, and only recently recognized category: is sleep.

Insufficient sleep (less than six hours per night) not only impairs neurobehavioral performance, but has been associated with increasing obesity and obesity-related diseases. The association between sleep shortage and excess weight is even stronger for children and adolescents. An important subset of people getting inadequate rest, and suffering metabolically, are those diagnosed with *obstructive sleep apnea.* Among adults without diabetes, increasing sleep apnea severity has been linked to rising blood sugar levels, and a higher risk of diabetes and cardiovascular disease. You don't have to have sleep apnea though to gain weight from missing sleep.

Sleep has a number of conflicting effects on metabolism. During sleep, we don't eat, and we aren't physically active. In other words, we have lower energy intake and expenditure, effects which would seem to offset each other. Lack of sleep, in turn, would logically convey those same offsetting effects in the opposite direction: more waking hours, more opportunity for both energy intake, and expenditure.

It gets complicated though.

For example, exhaustion reduces physical exertion. Sleep deprivation might, therefore, increase food intake (the time-and-opportunity factor) but reduce exercise (the exhaustion factor) thus promoting obesity.

The awake human expends energy three ways: (1) resting metabolism, (2) the *thermic effect of food* (calories burned during digestion), and (3) physical exercise. During sleep there is a lack of exercise, lack of food intake, and less metabolism—sleeping metabolic rate being 20 to 30 percent lower than awake resting metabolic rate. Therefore, all three energy-expenditure categories decline as one sleeps. Not sleeping, however, does not reverse the seemingly obesity-promoting effects of sleep. A whole raft of physiologic adaptations, triggered by sleep loss, are aimed at *increasing food intake* and *conserving energy*—both bad for the person trying to maintain or lower their BMI.

Specifically, sleep lack:

- *Dampens sympathetic nervous system tone.* Remember: we often try to counter the effects of insufficient sleep by consuming caffeine, a sympathetic nervous system stimulant. And many weight-loss drugs are caffeine-like/amphetamine-like stimulators, supporting in reverse the notion that hobbling sympathetic nervous system tone by sleep deprivation would be weight promoting.

- *Increases ghrelin*, a physiological appetite stimulant (I can vouch for this; staying up all night writing makes my appetite ravenous the next day).
- *Reduces resting metabolic rate*
- *Shifts metabolism away from fat*, toward carbohydrate burning, increasing hunger and food intake.
- *Reduces physical activity*

All of which adds up to, in the sleep-deprived organism, increased efficiency of fat storage and a sedentary lifestyle. In a paper titled "Update on Energy Homeostasis and Insufficient Sleep," in a 2012 *Journal of Clinical Endocrinology and Metabolism*, University of Chicago endocrinologist Plamen D. Penev stated this coordinated response favoring the intake and conservation of calories "may have evolved to offset the metabolic demands of extended wakefulness in natural habitats with limited food availability." Penev goes on to say, these effects could "be maladaptive in…a modern environment that allows many to overeat while maintaining a sedentary lifestyle without sufficient sleep."

It is thus clear that *enough sleep* needs to be elevated alongside *enough exercise* and *cutting calories* in the weight-management equation. In addition, any sleep disorders, such as sleep apnea, should be sought and treated as part of any serious effort to correct or avoid obesity, diabetes, and related conditions. Get thee to the sleep lab.

GET MENTAL?

I want to say a few words about another kind of exercise.

Intellectual.

An average man's brain oxidizes 120 grams of glucose per day, 25 percent of total energy expenditure, roughly the same as purposeful physical activity. And the brain almost exclusively uses glucose. Muscles use a mix of glucose, fats and ketone bodies. This means the brain, more than muscle, is exceptionally good at directly ridding the body of carbohydrates, before they can even think about being converted to and stocked away as fat.

Thus, to whatever extent increasing muscular physical activity contributes to effective weight management, it is my contention that increasing brain activity is at least equivalent. However, this is not an aspect of energy balance I've ever seen talked about, and even if "flexing one's noodle" (as my father used to say) has a relatively small effect on BMI (I think it may have a relatively large one), it is still a topic worth considering, along the lines of every little bit helps.

In support of this notion, I offer the well-established observation that obesity and obesity-related diseases afflict lower socioeconomic groups more than higher socioeconomic groups. There are a multitude of reasons, some of which we'll detail in a later chapter; however, a recent paper in *Diabetes Care*, looking specifically at socioeconomic impact on mortality in diabetes (to which obesity contributes), showed that if factors such as lack of access to quality medical care and psychological distress were filtered out, then *education level* (ranging from less than high school to college graduate or higher) and *financial wealth* (defined as owning stocks or a home) were both associated with the risk of death. That is, less education and a lack of wealth correlated with higher mortality. Interestingly, *income* did not contribute to mortality. Income being a parameter that can fluctuate, whereas wealth reflects ongoing financial factors and behaviors: savings habits, job stability, career advancement...

Accordingly—with respect to treating or avoiding obesity—I'd like to add the proposition that certain individuals, related to their years of education and type of occupation (managerial versus non-managerial, professional versus working class), might burn more glucose calories in the brain in an average day than others, who make their living in a more physically challenging manner.

Not to pick on particular occupations, but just to illustrate, the average university professor probably burns relatively more daily calories in the brain, compared to the average farm laborer, who probably burns more of his in working muscle. No disrespect to the laborer—but if excess intake of sugars are of particular concern in the modern obesity crisis (a topic to be developed later) there may be an advantage to brain metabolism directly and rapidly disposing of those calories, without need of insulin's help to do so by the way, as opposed to muscle metabolism which readily taps other resources, and requires insulin, under ordinary conditions, to use glucose.

I'm not suggesting the laborer might not have an IQ equal to the professor—intelligence and education are completely different propositions—but the nature of his or her work might make it less likely the laborer's IQ (that is, his or her brain metabolic potential) will be used to capacity in the course of an average day, unlike the professor's.

To emphasize, brain disposal of glucose, without need of insulin, may have advantages over muscle disposal of glucose, requiring insulin, in managing obesity. Why? Insulin can be thought of as the "stingy" hormone. It wants to store energy. It wants to hold back glucose and tuck it away as fat.

Muscle's greater need for insulin to get at the body's supply of sugar, therefore, makes it a less efficient disposer of sugar than the brain. And as we'll see later, anything that increases insulin levels, such as muscle glucose disposal, has the potential for promoting obesity: insulin being, in effect, a "fertilizer" for fat.

Obviously, many jobs are neither as physically taxing as farm laboring, nor as intellectually taxing as higher education. If you find yourself relatively sedentary throughout the workday, sitting behind a desk or at a computer station, doing fairly rote, perhaps boring tasks, then I urge you to choose leisure activities that exercise both the mind and the body. Accordingly, I recommend including activities in your life that challenge the brain, and minimizing those that don't:

- Read books, newspapers, magazines for entertainment and information in preference to passive options like TV, radio, DVDs.
- Computer and online activities vary: reading online for news and research should be as brain-stimulating as print materials; gaming is probably in the middle; and of course YouTube videos, and streaming movies and other programming are no better than TV.
- Play games
- Work puzzles, like the daily crossword in the newspaper.
- Cultivate a creative hobby.
- Take a course (a real one, or CD/DVD options).

6

DIET V. EXERCISE

The last couple of chapters suggested improving both nutritional and activity habits.

Which, however, is more important?

Nutrition—calories in?

Or exercise—calories out?

Both are valuable, and indiscretions, or limitations in one area can be offset by greater effort in the other. An injury, say, that limits physical exertion, might be made up for by greater calorie reduction. However, the real answer to the question depends on where one is in one's healthy BMI quest.

If you are at your desired BMI and you wish to maintain it, not yo-yo, not regain whatever you lost (the *maintenance phase*), then nutrition and activity are of roughly equal importance. If the goal is to maintain or improve musculoskeletal and cardiovascular fitness, conditioning, and endurance—a different kettle of fish from weight management, albeit a related kettle of fish—exercise is most important. Lastly, and this is the part most don't realize, if you are in the initial phase of weight loss (the *reduction phase*), exercise is *not* all that important. Nutrition is the bigger contributor to the calorie deficit that must occur for one to lose weight.

Now, I can't stress this enough, exercise is important. Don't misunderstand that. But if you decide you want to lose x number of pounds and you tell me that you're starting to jog in order to do that, without changing your diet, I'm going to tell you it probably isn't going to work. Exercise added to a reduced-calorie diet, may help, may improve the efficiency of your weight loss, but exercise alone—

unless you're running marathons—just doesn't burn enough extra calories for meaningful weight reduction. Running a mile, for example, only burns about a hundred calories, equal to a breakfast bar.

TYPE OF EXERCISE

Let's talk about the major varieties of exercise and how they differ with respect to health benefits. The two varieties are *resistance training* and *endurance training*.

Resistance training, aka weight training (i.e., weightlifting), and other forms of muscle-working exercise, such as yoga, and certain stretching exercises, increase strength and power, firm up bones and ligaments. Muscle mass is increased, especially in men, given the influence of testosterone. All these muscular size-, shape-, function-enhancing effects will benefit the individual's sense of well-being. The stronger, more limber you are, the better, more efficiently you will perform ordinary tasks: whether related to housework, or building construction.

Stronger, toned muscles improve posture and shore up joints, improving or preventing chronic pain syndromes related to arthritis and neuropathy. I experienced an epiphany about that from an interesting place. I married a horsewoman from way back, though at the time we met, Susan had been years away from riding. When I joined my practice in Tennessee, she fell in with a local physician equestrienne who generously allowed Susan use of her horse. Sometime later I made the mistake of (after one too many glasses of wine!) suggesting we buy a horse. Three horses and a farm later... but that's another story.

The point being, I was first exposed close-up to the magnificent athlete that is the domesticated horse some dozen odd years ago, and being a student of anatomy and physiology, I naturally gravitated toward that of the horse. When I contemplated its skeleton—built a model of one actually—I was struck that it seemed too structurally unstable to do what it did, support the animal through hauling, running at breakneck speeds, jumping, saddling loads on its back, and so forth. Form didn't seem to measure up to function. Then it occurred to me the skeleton, the bones and joints, didn't do those jobs alone. They had powerful tendons and that massive musculature to share the burden. Not just to move limbs and swivel joints, but to provide support, firm up the structure, knit the bones into proper anatomic position.

It didn't take much extrapolation for me to recognize the same was true of humans. Strong, toned muscles and tendons hold our bones in place, help support our joints and ligaments. Without that strength our joints are overstressed, pulled out of proper position—contributing to aches and pains and conditions like arthritis. Thus, careful strength training might treat and prevent musculoskeletal pain syndromes, in some cases, better than pain pills or joint injections.

Thicker muscles provide insulation, directly generate internal body heat, and literally provide padding, protecting against injury. Muscles store glycogen, a latticework of carbohydrate; the more muscular you are the more ready sources of glucose you can tap when blood sugar drops. I think this is why women tend to, in my experience, complain of "hypoglycemia" more than men, because they generally have less muscle, therefore less ready access to emergency carbohydrates. Interestingly, resistance exercise improves long-term blood-sugar control in type 1 diabetes better than aerobic exercise does.

Bottom line:

Resistance exercise to maintain and improve muscle size, strength, and tone is critical for a variety of reasons. Everybody should be doing it, regardless of age, to the best of their ability.

A lack of it may literally be crippling.

Now, to *endurance training*. Rather than stressing and loading muscle, endurance training involves physical activities that stress and load the heart and lungs, improving cardiovascular and cardiopulmonary fitness.

Also called *aerobic exercise*, endurance training generally consists of a lower level of exertion than weightlifting, but more sustained. A half-hour of walking or running, say, or bike-riding, or playing basketball, or using a treadmill or stationary bike: anything that gets the pulse up and keeps it up, and moves oxygen around the body. Better cardiovascular fitness leads to better stamina, making activities of daily living go easier, lowering the risk of death due to heart disease, and blood sugars in diabetics.

EXERCISE AND BMI REDUCTION

Regular physical activity, of different varieties, is important for a whole host of reasons. It is not, however, particularly important for the reduction phase of weight management, as I've said. Calorie reduction, reduced energy intake, is far more important. For example, a 1988 paper in the *New England Journal of Medicine* showed over one year a mean weight loss of 9 pounds in a group participating only in exercise, and 16 pounds in one receiving only a dietary prescription.

Why?

Of total daily energy expenditure, *only about 15 percent is voluntary physical activity*. The rest goes to generating internal body heat (another 15 percent) and basal metabolism (70 percent), which is the energy expenditure resulting from the heart beating and lungs breathing and brain thinking and every other organ and system operating in a person seated at rest. In fact, resting skeletal muscle is a remarkably large contributor to basal metabolism, which will become important in the next subchapter when we talk about weight maintenance. In other words, muscle is a very important disposer of calories, a very important factor on the energy expenditure side of the energy-balance equation—and therefore, having more muscle, promoted by certain types of exercise, is important to energy balance—but it is *resting* muscle, not *exercising* muscle that has the greater impact.

Exercise just doesn't add that much directly, doesn't bring that much to the table, if you'll pardon the pun.

The percentages cited above are obviously averages. Calories allocated to physical activity are greater in more athletic individuals. In marathon runners, or those undergoing military training, calories consumed by exercise might be a significant percentage of the total, but most of us aren't doing anything close to that, even those of us going to some effort.

Say I'm average and 15 percent of my 2000 calories per day are burned by physical exertion. And say I'm ten pounds overweight and decide to start jogging to lose those ten pounds. Say the increased exercise doubles the portion of my total calorie expenditure due to activity. That means 30 percent of my daily calories burned go to exercise; for every 100 calories I eat, 30 vaporizes in physical exertion. But 15 of those were already doing so, before the additional exercise, when I was staying ten pounds overweight. My new effort is burning an additional 15 of every 100 calories eaten. If I don't change my diet, stay at 2000 calories per day—*how long to lose the ten pounds?*

It takes a deficit of 3500 calories to lose one pound. Thus, to lose ten pounds takes a deficit of 35,000 calories (35,000 calories more burned than swallowed). If my added exercise gets me there at a rate of 15 calories per 100, that's 300 calories per 2000 of daily intake. If we divide the needed 35,000-calorie deficit by the 300 per day from extra exercise, that's almost 120 days (35,000 ÷ 300 = 116.667).

Four months to lose 10 pounds.

If I double my daily physical activity and never miss a day.

That is something, of course, and I wouldn't discourage it, except to counsel that the effort might not match the benefit and might lead to a flagging of interest and motivation.

More Reflections on the 3500-Calorie Rule

It has already been noted that running a mile burns about 100 calories. Thus, the number of calories burned by exercise isn't that much relative to the 3500-calorie deficit required to lose just one pound. To accomplish that deficit with running alone requires 35 miles of running. That's five miles per day, each and every day, to lose one pound per week. Can you do that?

Not me.

Recent papers even challenge the "3500-calorie rule" as *over*estimating the impact of exercise over long periods of time. The source of the discrepancy lies in the fact that every unit of weight we lose lessens the number of calories burned by equal amounts of exercise. A person walking a mile per day might be predicted to lose 50 pounds in five years under the 3500 rule, but would in fact only lose 10 pounds.

Nutritional modification is absolutely necessary for meaningful BMI lowering. Physical activity contributes, and has many other benefits—including mitigating health-damaging effects of obesity, and perhaps putting to healthier use hours in the day that might otherwise be spent eating and watching TV—but weight loss itself is not the most robust of these benefits.

EXERCISE AND BMI MAINTENANCE

Okay. We've lost the weight we wanted. How do we maintain it, avoid the diet rollercoaster? Exercise is important for *maintaining* a reduced BMI, and maintenance is as important as loss, because *there really isn't any point to losing weight you're going to gain right back*. Therefore, in spite of anything else said, exercise must not be ignored in any serious effort at body-weight management.

The reason physical activity is specifically important to BMI maintenance relates to the subconscious signals from the brain's appetite centers, telling us when we're full, and when we're hungry. We need to be able to depend on satiety (fullness) because it is simply impossible—or, anyway, highly impractical and improbable—to day in, day out, year after year, consciously monitor and regulate calorie intake. The effort fails and BMI increases. How do we enhance the effectiveness of these automatic signals saying, "Don't eat any more, you'll gain weight," or "Do eat more, you're losing weight"?

Can you guess?

Activity.

Exercise. The brain regulates our ins and outs better, more accurately, at a high average exertion level, compared to a sedentary level.

Also, skeletal muscle, in addition to burning calories during exercise, also burns a lot of calories at rest. Taken as a whole, the musculature of the human body is probably its largest organ. And resistance training increases the mass of that large organ, which increases its calorie consumption at rest. In other words, resistance training increasing muscle mass also increases basal metabolic rate, which reduces, or at least attenuates increases in fat mass. Thus, I would argue that resistance training is likely more important to obesity treatment than endurance training, although both have an important place in a healthy lifestyle.

And by the way, it occurs to me, many of my patients over the years, in talking about their weight-management efforts, especially women, have included a concern about adding too much muscle. Specifically they are worried that they are going to weigh more on the bathroom scale if they add muscle.

Maybe they will.

I don't care.

In managing obesity and preventing obesity-related disease, we don't care about anything other than fat. Period. Nothing else. Not water weight, certainly not muscle. In fact, assuming it was accumulated naturally—not via anabolic steroids, or growth-hormone shots, and so forth—I'm not sure that there is any muscle-mass accumulation I would consider to be a bad thing. The more the merrier, and if there are people out there attenuating their weight-loss efforts out of concern for "adding muscle weight," I would just chalk that up to yet another myth or misconception hampering effective management of the obesity epidemic.

THE LESS YOU DO TODAY...

There are diseases my orthopedic, rheumatology, and PMR (pain management/rehabilitation) colleagues deal with that afflict patients with inordinate physical pain exacerbated by exercise. Fibromyalgia would be an example, and various musculoskeletal strain syndromes, like tendonitis. I don't suggest anyone violate doctor's orders regarding any activity restrictions appropriate to those diagnoses; however, if anyone ever told me to avoid some significant physical activity for a prolonged period, I'd be asking a lot of questions. I'm not counting, obviously, recovery from a major fracture, or major joint surgery, or serious rheumatic diseases, like rheumatoid arthritis, but I have often admonished my patients: "The less you do today, the less you'll be able to do a year from now."

Different subject, but the worse thing I ever saw a doctor do was put my late mother on a restricted diet (specifically, a diverticulosis diet, avoiding seeds and such) because it started her down a path of neurotic nutritional, and eventually physical invalidity. I hate putting—I think I can honestly say I never have put—a patient on any long-term physical restriction. Granted, as an endocrinologist, I don't much deal with physical problems, and the problems I do deal with, like diabetes, typically benefit from activity, rather than the opposite. Of course, restricting "unhealthy" dietary habits are part and parcel of my practice, but as you'll see, I'm more liberal than most even on that.

My point is, humans—whether robust 18-year-old men or frail 70-year-old ladies—were meant to be physically active, and suffer from lack of it, obesity being but one of the potential negative consequences. Be physical. Look for ways to be physical, rather than for ways to avoid it, and don't be scared off, within reason, by discomfort.

Everybody hurts somewhere, from time to time. And certainly everybody hurts who does something physical that they're not used to, pushing the envelope of their musculoskeletal fitness. They get sore muscles. That's normal physiology, and after a period of rest, the same activity, repeated, should result in less, or hopefully no pain.

That's called *conditioning.*

Conditioning is good.

Not unusually I see patients—generally older women, a demographic less likely to have been socialized from an early age toward physical activity (my mother thought physical exertion unladylike)—who report that exercise, perhaps just walking, causes pain and therefore they can't exercise. They might've been diagnosed with fibromyalgia, and that might be proper, or they might've just had that label pasted on them, and what they really have is *chronic poor conditioning.*

The answer to which is rest, followed by repeating the offending activity, and keep repeating it with increasing intensity and duration, until the pain returns, then give it another rest. If there is real disease, the situation might or might not improve. But chronic poor conditioning will. I think everybody in that boat should try what I'm suggesting, perhaps before visiting the doctor, because nothing will cure chronic poor conditioning except regular physical activity.

No medicine will help.

Why Take a Pill?

I also discourage pain relievers, prescriptions or over-the-counter, for musculoskeletal pain caused by simple exertion. If the pain isn't suggesting a serious disease or injury, but part of normal physiology, why take a drug that could have side effects? Possibly serious side effects. Most nonsteroidal anti-inflammatory drugs (NSAIDs), like ibuprofen, can damage the kidneys and the lining of the stomach. Certainly, were I going to use an NSAID for exercise-induced soreness, I would only take one or two doses.

Why take any?

Why risk side effects, when the pain will be self-limited (doctor-speak for, *it'll get better on it's own*)? Why medicate minor pain? We are an overmedicated society, obsessed with comfort and convenience and that is part of the cause of the epidemic of obesity, and another consequence of that obsession is the notion that we are supposed to go through life pain free, that we aren't supposed to have to put up with anything. My advice: put up with it. Everybody has a sore knee or backache from time to time and it usually gets better—but we never realize it gets better because we take a pill and assume the pill is what helped.

Other than avoiding side effects and saving a few pennies, might there be other reasons to "put up with" minor pain?

I believe so.

Pain is the body's natural warning sign.

If something hurts, it's damaged. If something causes pain, it's doing damage. The very last thing we should be doing is medicating pain for the purpose of continuing the activity that inflicted the pain, the damage, in the first place. My advice above was to rest the sore muscle, until it heals, then rechallenge it. Typically the same level of activity will be better tolerated, or perhaps you will take it easier, or be more careful, the next time around. Taking a pill though, to deaden the pain—blind ourselves to the warning sign—then continuing the damaging activity could worsen the injury to the point it does need medical treatment, even to the point it becomes chronic, debilitating, perhaps requiring more and stronger painkillers.*

And since this is a book about obesity—and I freely acknowledge this part of the discussion colors way outside the lines of my expertise as an endocrinologist—I will tie those postulated "more and stronger painkillers" back to our main topic of obesity. Steroids are commonly prescribed for all kinds of pain syndromes, ranging from acute to chronic, and steroids promote weight gain. (An occasional week of a tapering "steroid burst" is not going to significantly alter ones weight management, and can be very helpful in the right situation, to which I can personally attest, but beyond that, steroids for pain should be avoided if possible.) Another example: Lyrica, prescribed for certain chronic pain situations, causes drowsiness, which might lessen activity, promoting obesity.

Another reason to avoid medicating minor pain related to overexertion? And this is a little metaphysical—pain is a perception. It is a neuro-electro-chemical signal traveling from the periphery to the brain via nerves, but how the conscious mind registers and reacts to it is highly variable. We all know the stereotype of the seriously wounded soldier fighting on bravely, unmindful of grave injuries. What might be slight discomfort to one, might seem crippling to another. I think—and this is pure speculation on my part—if we avoid treating minor pain we might train our consciousness and subconsciousness to perceive pain less severely. If we let things progress naturally, we might accept and internalize the notion that pain often gets better on its own, then the pain itself might be seem less severe from the get-go. And if we think of sore muscles as "badges of honor" for accomplishing a particular intensity and duration of exertion, rather than as an injury or illness to be treated,

---

* I acknowledge this piece of advice might seem naïve at best, unsympathetic, even elitist at worst, applied to the person who, say, lifts crates for a living, getting a resulting backache. It's nice to tell that person to lay off the activity, rather than take a pill to keep doing the activity, except that the activity in the example is providing that person's livelihood. There is no ideal answer to a lot of situations—I'm merely suggesting an approach that might not otherwise be thought of.

again I think they might not be regarded as severely.

Let nature take its course. I'm not one who believes everything "natural" is necessarily better or safer, but there is some truth in that notion. And what could be more natural than allowing a bicep made sore by heavy lifting to improve at it own pace without intervention?

The point is to be as active as possible, for many reasons, including maintaining a healthy weight. Push for the opportunity and ability to exert yourself, because to not, to give into pain, for example, will hobble your weight-management efforts, and increase your risk of obesity-associated disease. And if you are in the unfortunate position of having to restrict your activity over an extended period, due say to a serious injury, or perhaps even permanently due to a serious musculoskeletal or neurological disability, then you will as a consequence have more difficulty maintaining or achieving a healthy weight, and following the best diet possible becomes even more critical.

7

DON'T PIT YOUR WEIGHT LOSS AGAINST OTHERS'

A social-support network is good. If you are struggling to establish and maintain a healthier lifestyle to reduce your BMI and risk of cardiovascular disease and death, it is good to have people to talk to about that struggle. They might offer advice or insight, or make you accountable, make you feel guilty if you cheat. If two of you are trying you can be supportive and encouraging of each other. Some weight-loss programs involve group meetings and public weigh-ins, in which successes are applauded, failures consoled.

However, you must absolutely forget about comparing other's weight-loss successes with your perceived failures. Do not punish or criticize yourself because you aren't losing as fast or as much as somebody else. A wise person once said: "The only person you'll ever have to be better than is the person you were yesterday."

Nowhere is that more true than with body weight.

Comparisons to others are complete folly.

I heard a pastor once on the radio say: "Never compare your insides to anybody else's outsides."

(He wasn't talking about weight, but the statement is apropos.)

Nevertheless, I cannot begin to count how many patients I've had bemoaning the fact that they have done exactly the same things as another person, yet that other person has lost x pounds and they haven't. To make matters worse, often, my patient is a young woman, and the other person is her male significant other, husband or boyfriend.

METABOLIC INEQUALITY

First, you are utterly lying to yourself if you believe you're eating, drinking, and exercising exactly the same as any other person, and deluding yourself if you're expecting to match any other person's weight-management outcomes. Consider: exactly the same number of grams of bread and lunch meat, and so on, and so on, consumed every day; exact same number of steps walked every day; exact same basal metabolic rate to start with, which accounts for 60 to 70 percent of daily energy usage, and which varies significantly with gender, body weight, height and age.* Put simply, those criteria will never be met. Your daily energy expenditure—barring the remotest coincidence—will never equal that of any other person; therefore even if you were eating, drinking, and exercising *exactly* the same (just as remote a possibility), your energy balances still would differ.

This is not a discussion worth having—it's ridiculous—and yet I have it virtually every day. People really believe they are doing the same thing as somebody who is losing weight and therefore there is something wrong with them that needs to be fixed (that I need to fix, and they're upset when I say I can't) because they aren't losing a similar amount of weight as the other person.

Your weight management has nothing to do with anyone else's.

Gender Impacts Metabolism

The above is especially true if we're talking about spouses, or more generally, men and women. There are inequities. Men and women were not created equal, not biologically. The differences, most of you

---

* The Harris-Benedict Formula determines basal metabolic rate, aka basal energy expenditure (BEE), as follows:
- Male BEE = 66 + (13.7 x CIBW in kilograms[kg]) + (5 x Height in centimeters) - (6.8 x Age in years)
- Female BEE = 655 + (9.6 x CIBW) + (1.7 x Height) - (4.7 x Age)
- Where CIBW is "corrected ideal body weight," also calculated differently (see below) for men versus women, as is ideal body weight (IBW) itself. Don't get bogged down in any of these equations, just note the differences.
  - o Male IBW = 50kg for the first 5ft of height + 2.3kg for each 1in > 5ft
  - o Female IBW = 45.5kg for the first 5ft + 2.3kg per 1in > 5ft
  - o Male CIBW = IBW + 0.3 x (actual weight - IBW)
  - o Female CIBW = IBW + 0.25 x (actual weight - IBW)

know, boil down to levels of the two major sex steroids, *testosterone* and *estrogen*. Actually several hormones perform estrogenic functions, and several perform androgenic, or testosterone-like actions. I won't complicate the discussion by naming those other hormones; I will simply refer to testosterone and estrogen in general terms, both of which can be found in both sexes, in different amounts. The average testosterone concentration in male blood is 20 fold greater than in a female sample; whereas reproductive-age women have 40 fold greater circulating estrogen concentrations compared to men.

Testosterone

Testosterone, literally, makes the man. All human embryos start out anatomically female and remain female unless something intervenes. That something is the Y chromosome and the genetically male fetus's own testosterone, which trigger the formation of male anatomy. Later, during puberty, testosterone triggers secondary sexual characteristics, such as growth of the external genitalia, and appearance of facial and body hair. Testosterone promotes enlargement of the kidneys and liver in men, and stimulates bone-marrow red-blood-cell production. Testosterone, interacting with locally produced estrogen in the brain, shapes stereotypically male behavior patterns, including physical aggressiveness. Lastly, skeletal muscle is an important target of testosterone, producing some of the most striking of the physical differences between the sexes. In short, higher testosterone in men promotes the growth of internal organs, and other functioning tissues, such as bone marrow, and especially bigger and stronger muscles, all at the expense of body fat.

Any calories shunted to these burgeoning tissues will not be available to be stored as fat within *adipose tissue*. Thus, testosterone opposes the laying down of excess fat. Further, the characteristic behavioral effect of testosterone, a tendency towards aggressiveness, which might serve society well in hunter-gatherer or war-fighting situations—and perhaps ill in other arenas—may promote a drive in some men to be more athletic, to engage in physical activity of greater intensity and duration, relative to women of comparable age and health. Obviously I speak of a hypothetical average man and woman. As they say, individual results may vary; many women are, for example, far more athletic than I.

Estrogen

Estrogen dominance in women promotes growth and function of the female reproductive tract, and feminine secondary sexual characteristics, including localized fat deposition in the breast, buttock, and hip areas. Either through direct estrogen action, or a paucity of testosterone—resulting in the converse of all testosterone's effects listed above—women have a higher percentage of body fat than men of matching age and BMI.

All this goes in support of pregnancy and motherhood. It benefits the growing fetus and nursing infant for the mother to have a ready supply of stored energy—fat—from which to provide sustenance. As well, greater quantities of subcutaneous fat (fat under the skin) lay the foundation, literally, for that stereotypical feminine softness, and roundness of features, which proffers the infant warmth and protection from the elements and other threats. Estrogen, among its many other effects, causes the liver to produce a protein (*sex-hormone binding globulin*) that binds testosterone in the blood, making that hormone less readily available. Also, more fat means more aromatase, an enzyme contained in adipose tissue that converts testosterone to estrogen. Thus, estrogen through several mechanisms deliberately depletes the female body of testosterone's effects.

The upshot of it all being that men have a normal physiology favoring, and may more likely engage in behaviors favoring, a lower percentage of body fat, and greater ease of weight loss. *All other things being equal, most men will have an easier time losing weight than most women.*

Therefore, women should never—*repeat, never*—compare weight-loss successes and failures to that of men. The results will not be helpful, and will cause unwarranted frustration.

This is a deck stacked against women.

Why?

DR. RONE'S POLITICALLY INCORRECT PET THEORY

Women are programmed to hold onto excess weight more tenaciously than men for reasons which are, I believe, sociobiological and anthropological...

In prehistory, and in the early medieval dark ages, and even later in all but the most highly ordered segments of society—the upper strata in, say, a large city or town—life was hard, very difficult. There were physical dangers, risks of attack, constant threats of poverty and famine. The men most likely to survive to father multiple offspring, who would be most likely to survive into adulthood and pass along their paternal genes to a third generation, were the men who were genetically programmed to produce higher testosterone levels, resulting in heavier muscle mass, greater strength and stamina, and enhanced aggressiveness. These men would be better hunters and gatherers, by which they provided necessities to their families, and they would be more likely to prevail when defending home and hearth against wild predators, or rival marauding humans.

Women, in turn, in these primitive and pre-modern societies, were more likely to bear more children, who survived into adulthood to pass along their mothers' genes, if they were genetically programmed to store a lot of fat in times of plenty, so that even in the lean times they were able to conceive and carry a pregnancy to term, and nourish the infant through its vulnerable early life. The importance of adiposity to reproduction is readily evidenced today by women who have low body fat percentages (owing to, say, anorexia nervosa, or training as an elite-level gymnast or runner) losing their menses and becoming infertile.

> "But Cliff, it'll be so terrible. I'll, I'll be so cold and all alone. Who will keep me warm?"
>
> "You'll do fine Margaret. Women have that extra layer of fat."
>
> —*Cheers* TV episode, 1989

Nor should we dismiss the biological value of feminine "softness" and "roundness." I mention this not for titillation purposes, but in fact, an infant or young child who more strongly sought and received the comfort and protection of its mother's body would be more likely to survive a harsh environment. And, to the extent the characteristic female body-fat morphology bestows a shape and texture men find arousing, women with a greater percentage body fat would be better able to attract mates and have more babies to propagate their genes.

I believe this situation—wherein survival depended directly upon male strength and female nurturing—continued for most human societies through the industrial revolution, and analogous challenges (poverty, disease), leading to similar evolutionary pressures, continued even until the latter half of the 20th century, even in the United States and Western Europe.

Under this scenario, throughout much of human history natural selection has favored the survival and propagation of—to be blunt—

men who tended toward leanness, and women who tended toward fatness.

This is a chauvinistic take on history, I'll grant you, and I'm generalizing and simplifying. I am neither historian nor anthropologist. But I think my scenario forges a generally accurate, if superficial, impression of the genetic pressures that might have created the gender dimorphism observable today, the weight-management inequity between men and women.

I'll carry this argument a step further:

I recall an editorial in a major endocrinology journal in the last few years titled, "The Fall of Testosterone," and I've attended a symposium on the same subject.

Testosterone levels in men are not as high on average as once they were.

One postulated explanation is the epidemic of obesity. Fat contains *aromatase* that converts testosterone to estrogen. Any man that has a higher percentage body fat also has more aromatase, and likely a lower testosterone level, and higher estrogen level. Experts have not felt, however, that higher average BMIs completely explain the observed testosterone decline.

I believe an extrapolation of my caveman theory might contribute to understanding why testosterone levels are dropping.

If in the Stone Age brawn trumped brains—the man with more brawn than intellect was better able to support and protect his home, propagate his family—then natural selection would favor brawn, and the higher testosterone levels that produce brawn.

Gradually, as technology and social order advanced, the need for physical prowess to survive lessened. Certainly this has been a gradual process. The early 20th century farmer in the United States probably did not often have need to engage in physical combat with predatory wildlife or human evildoers, but he still had to do backbreaking work, day in and day out, to support his family.

In the last fifty years, especially the last ten or twenty, there have been huge shifts in the Western economies towards more intellectual professions, away from physically challenging ones. In other words, today, in our digital-, information-, electronic-age, brains trump brawn.

I'm not saying a muscularly endowed man can't also be an intellectual dynamo, but since both aren't necessary for survival and childrearing anymore, greater multitudes of less-brawny types are out there making good livings with flourishing families, propagating those less-brawny genes. I believe that for the past dozen or two generations in Western societies we have seen the dilution of a gene pool once chockfull of traits favoring high testosterone, with genes that promote lower testosterone (which, while not necessarily an advantage, is no longer the disadvantage it once was). And I think that dilution has progressed exponentially in the past couple of generations—hence, the "fall" of testosterone.

8

NON-GENDER METABOLIC VARIABLES

Gender is only one factor making one person's weight management easier or harder than another's. As stated previously, we all have different facial structures and hair colors and personalities—and metabolisms. Some metabolic variations arise from normal physiology, some from pathology, and in some cases the line between physiology and disease may only be a matter of degree.

INSULIN RESISTANCE AND DIABETES

As most are aware, *diabetes mellitus* is a condition in which glucose levels in the bloodstream ("blood sugars") run chronically high to a degree sufficient to damage organs, including the eyes, kidneys, and nerves. This sixth greatest cause of death due to disease in the U.S. in 2010, and ninth in the world, exists in several forms, by far the most common of which, and the form most connected to obesity is Type 2 diabetes mellitus (T2DM). Once upon a time known as "adult-onset diabetes," T2DM occurs far too commonly in youth these days to continue going by that nomenclature. T2DM is a *polygenic* disorder, meaning multiple *genotypes* (individual genes) coalesce to form the *phenotype* (the observable properties) that we see as T2DM. The more "diabetogenic" genes a person is born with, the more likely he or she is to develop diabetes, and the earlier it is likely to happen. A person is at roughly twice the risk whose mother and father both had diabetes, compared to only one parent.

The genes causing T2DM, to put this very simply, are those affecting insulin production and sensitivity. *Insulin* is the hormone produced by the pancreas that lowers blood glucose. It is the only substance in the body, in fact, to lower blood glucose, while many work to increase it. (An elegant design feature, by the way, if you think about it: given that an accidental low blood sugar can cause instant death, whereas higher blood sugars prevent the former, and while they are not always good, if too high, the harm they can do is very slow to accumulate, compared to that instant-death thing.) Insulin triggers events that transport glucose from the blood to the interior of cells, muscle cells, for example. *Insulin sensitivity* is the term describing how efficiently this shuttling of glucose takes place, an important metabolic consideration because glucose must find itself inside a cell before it can ever be subject to cellular metabolism, resulting for example in it being burned (or *oxidized*) to yield energy.

If one's pancreas must produce twice as much insulin as "normal" to clear the glucose from a meal out of the blood, that person is said to be half as insulin sensitive as normal. Or, twice as *insulin resistant.*

Usually we talk about insulin resistance as if it were a bad thing. Insulin resistance is, however, advantageous during famines because it limits the wasting of calories in times of plenty, promoting their storage in the form of fat, whereupon they are burned at some future point when food is scarce—when there is a potato famine, or one is interned in a concentration camp. Since neither eventuality, nor anything similar, is likely to befall us in present-day America or the rest of the developed world, genes for insulin resistance, which once had a positive role, are today more likely to have a negative impact, leading to excess fat storage, obesity, and full-blown T2DM.

Thus, insulin-resistance genes, promoting survival during nutritional stress, can be thought of as a *physiologically normal beneficial genetic variant.* A metabolic emergency-preparedness system, so to speak. Too many such genes, though, concentrated in one person, results in diabetes and all its risks, including blindness, kidney failure, neuropathic pain or numbness, amputation, heart disease, and death. Clearly the latter is a disease—*pathology*, not *physiology*—yet the demarcation is blurred.

Any degree of insulin resistance, which most Americans probably possess in some measure, excluding perhaps those seeming to remain skinny no matter what they eat—and those people do exist, that's no myth—promotes the deposition of fat and resists its loss. The more genes for insulin resistance you inherited from your parents, then, the more difficult managing your weight will be.

Diabetics really do have stronger appetites, by the way, than non-diabetics, which is part of the difficulty getting their blood sugars under control, and regulating their weight. This feature of diabetes is related to the lack of or resistance to a variety of other hormones besides insulin, which is the one that gets all the attention. These other hormones are involved in the appetite and fullness signals between the GI tract and brain, and include *amylin*, produced by the pancreas, and GLP-1, released by the small intestine. Lastly, it was noted in Chapter 2 that insulin, not to be outdone, also travels to the brain and shuts off appetite. And like the rest of the body, the brain in T2DM is insulin resistant, meaning in this instance, resistant to appetite suppression.

Thus, if you have diabetes, or a strong family history of it, several perturbations will make it harder than average for you to lose weight. You might have even been telling your doctors this for years, falling on deaf ears, since much of this pathophysiology has only recently been worked out—a tragic irony, since good BMI management is key to treating diabetes and preventing its complications.

Incidentally, in her paper, "Diabetes: Have We Got it All Wrong?"—subtitled "Insulin Hypersecretion and Food Additives: Cause of Obesity and Diabetes?"—in the December 2012 *Diabetes Care*, Barbara Corkey, Ph.D. of Boston University proposes that genetics-driven insulin resistance is not the foundational defect in T2DM that most doctors and researchers feel it to be. She postulates that fats, proteins, artificial sweeteners, and other environmental toxins, make insulin release inappropriately high relative to the amount of glucose in the bloodstream. In order for this *hyperinsulinemia* to not trigger dangerous hypoglycemia (low blood sugar), Dr. Corkey proposes that insulin resistance might be a beneficial adaptation, rather than the "cause" of T2DM.

As my interpretation of the theory goes, against the background described above, other environmental pollutants, such as bisphenol A, commonly used in food and beverage containers, and perhaps additional genes that hobble insulin release, would then lead to diabetes in the face of this "beneficial adaptive insulin resistance."

This is an area of ongoing research but if it turns out to be even partly true, it bolsters the proposition I espouse that the obesity and diabetes epidemics are consequences of a "toxic" environment of food additives, and marketing, and public-educational misdirection, at least as much, perhaps more so, than they are consequences of overindulgence and idleness.

Furthermore, if Corkey's alternative model of diabetes is borne out, we are witnessing what science philosopher Thomas S. Kuhn called, in 1962, a "crisis." A scientific crisis, in Kuhn's view, occurs when prevailing scientific dogma (in this case, the paradigm that genetic insulin resistance is the fundamental trigger for diabetes) is challenged—which may lead to a "revolution," and the eventual adoption of a new "paradigm" (see Appendix B).

THYROID HORMONE AND VICIOUS CYCLING

The thyroid is the largest pure endocrine gland in humans. A thyroid gland is found in every vertebrate species, from fish, to lizards, to mammals. In adult humans the thyroid gland receives, gram for gram, 50 percent more blood flow than the kidneys. All suggesting the thyroid gland is important. (Despite my cardiologist friend's quip: "When the thyroid fails, they don't call it the big one.")

There are three common (mis?)perceptions about the thyroid and its product, thyroid hormone, which are overblown by patients, and under-blown by their doctors. The first of these is that thyroid hormone is a key regulator of body weight, the second, thyroid deficiency, *hypothyroidism*, is a major cause of human obesity, and third, thyroid-replacement therapy, in whatever form, is an effective and safe way to lose weight.

Thyroid hormone is, to be sure, a primary regulator of metabolism, especially metabolism devoted to generating internal body heat. It sets the body's idle speed, its metabolic rate. Too little thyroid hormone makes us fatigued and lethargic, depressed perhaps. The skin thickens and dries. We feel cold, don't think as fast, organ systems operate sluggishly, producing any number of a long list of symptoms. And, yes, there is weight gain—how much is debatable, but to argue that hypothyroidism doesn't affect weight is absurd. Look no further than the opposite disease—*hyperthyroidism*—a classic symptom of which is weight loss despite a preserved appetite, calories wasted owing to an overly exuberant metabolism. Surely then hypothyroidism promotes the opposite effect? Indeed, it does; however, the quantity of weight gain solely due to hypothyroidism seems relatively small. Ten pounds is oft quoted, though I'm not sure where that comes from. A 2005 Danish paper in the *Journal of Clinical Endocrinology and Metabolism* compared obesity rates in people whose thyroid levels were low-normal versus those who were high-normal.

The low-normal-thyroid group *was* twice as likely to be obese. However, everybody in the study gained weight. No thyroid level anywhere between the physiological extremes prevented weight gain; weight gain is human nature, in other words. And the average weight difference between the worst group in the Danish study and the best group was only nine pounds!

Further confusing things, there is recent work suggesting that obesity might actually cause hypothyroidism, as opposed to hypothyroidism causing obesity, the theory being that the chronic low-grade inflammation associated with obesity promotes an immune-system attack on the thyroid gland.* Which came first, in other words, the chicken or the egg?

It does seem fair to say that some weight gain results from hypothyroidism, and it is reasonable to assume more severe hypothyroidism has a greater impact. Thyroid dysfunction, however, is not the sole cause of morbid obesity in a person weighing, say, 300 pounds. It is a contributor, perhaps, not the cause.

That said—hypothyroidism definitely produces a whole raft of other problems that of their own accord promote weight gain. Hypothyroidism hobbles the metabolism and function of every tissue, every organ. Might those dysfunctional organs augment whatever weight gain is caused by a dysfunctional thyroid gland? Might they further tilt the energy-intake/energy-expenditure equation toward the fat-storage side? And if it is true that weight gain begets hypothyroidism and hypothyroidism begets, to at least some degree, weight gain, then there could be some serious vicious cycling in play.

Fatigue

Hypothyroidism causes fatigue.

A heart not pumping as vigorously, because of hypothyroidism, will cause more fatigue, and a muscle not extracting enough energy from fuel available, because of hypothyroidism, will cause more fatigue, and a liver that cannot break down toxins as efficiently, because of hypothyroidism, will cause more fatigue, and so on. Fatigue limits exercise, begetting more fatigue via poor cardiovascular and musculoskeletal conditioning. And of course, inadequate exercise makes it harder to maintain or lose weight. And if you don't spend your leisure hours exercising, you might be eating.

---

* *Autoimmunity*, one's own immune system attacking the body, is a common cause of thyroid disease in the United States.

Depression

Hypothyroidism causes depression.

Depressed people tend to have more unhealthy body fat. Why? That's a question for researchers, but it is certainly not hard to speculate. Some depressed people have an increased appetite. Depression may cause insomnia, sleep lack promoting weight gain, as we've discussed, as well as being yet another energy sapper. Depressed patients lose interest or pleasure in usual activities, which might limit one's activity, and exercise intensity. Body movements are slowed; the person may be indecisive. These are but a few manifestations of depression, which I selected for mention as plausible weight-gain triggers. Then of course, depressed people might be treated with psychotropic medications, many of which cause weight gain, including tricyclic antidepressants, monoamine oxidase inhibitors, some newer antidepressants, lithium, and the atypical antipsychotics.

Other Thyroid Effects

Musculoskeletal symptoms, stiffness and soreness, occur in hypothyroidism, limiting activity. Constipation is common, and though increased stool retention has nothing to do with true obesity, retained fecal material does contain water and other matter, adding weight measured on the bathroom scale. For that matter, hypothyroidism is associated with fluid retention in the skin, and might promote congestive heart failure, which causes weight gain due to fluid and salt overload.

Hypothyroidism, in summary, slows the body's utilization of energy resources, and brings on a host of other effects that cause fatigue, or otherwise limit physical activity. All interfering with calorie burning. In other words, hypothyroidism mostly affects the energy-expenditure side of the energy-balance equation. That's an important observation relating to how much hypothyroidism might contribute to a weight problem, or how much an increase in thyroid levels might contribute to solving that problem.

We've said that modifying the calories-out side—exercising more, for example—doesn't do all that much for actual weight loss; it isn't as important as reducing calorie intake (recalling the "3500 rule"— that a 3500-calorie deficit is needed to lose one pound, and that kind of deficit is hard to achieve with exercise alone). Therefore, since hypothyroidism mostly hobbles voluntary physical activity, its effect on initial weight loss might not be that dramatic. In fact, it's probably fair to say thyroid status, like exercise, impacts *weight maintenance* more than one's ability to lose weight to begin with.

Does hypothyroidism affect energy intake?

Perhaps. Appetite stimulation is sometimes seen in depression, and the mental sluggishness associated with hypothyroidism—"brain fog," some call it—might impair one's focus on, and commitment to nutritional modifications.

Everybody is different. Every obese person has a different combination of causes and solutions for their unhealthy weight. In some people hypothyroidism is one of those causes, affecting mostly energy expenditure, but in some cases energy intake as well. Depending on how many other things are going on, how effectively they are being dealt with, treating the thyroid problem might have either a significant or negligible impact on one's weight management. It is clear to me though that thyroid status should be considered, and I think too often it isn't by physicians.

Bottom line:

There is no reason hypothyroid people can't lose weight if they cut calorie intake to less than the number of calories burned (and, lest I sound too Pollyannaish, recalling that the calories-burned figure is highly changeable, and largely out of our voluntary control; it's a little like aiming at a moving target wearing a blindfold, matching intake to expenditure). But all of that is the same challenge everyone has, regardless of thyroid status. Now, because fewer calories are liable to be burned by the hypothyroid person, weight loss might be more difficult, might require a greater reduction in calories, but it is not the impossibility of myth. Hypothyroidism doesn't create or destroy matter either. The other challenge, though, often the bigger one, everyone has regardless of thyroid status is weight maintenance, following loss. And thyroid hormone may well have a very significant role in that phase of weight control.

I'm going to toss, at this juncture, some pure speculation onto the grill of our discussion of hypothyroidism and weight management. It was stated in Chapter 2 that energy balance in humans in complex and regulated and involves a *set point*, like a thermostat setting, around which the brain works to maintain a certain weight, even if that set-point weight is 350 pounds. Any truly effective obesity treatment must lower that set point. What if correcting a thyroid deficiency, even if only a mild one, is enough of a "shock" to the system to be one of those set-point lowering factors that are needed for meaningful weight management. Were that the case, a thyroid pill alone would not be enough to reduce weight, but a combination of a thyroid pill and healthy lifestyle modifications involving nutrition and physical activity might well be a very potent weight-loss combination, as I have had occasion to observe.

Accordingly, as a thyroidologist (my primary calling), I do consider starting treatment with, or increasing an existing dose of thyroid hormone in those having unusual difficulty managing weight, if I think a lack of thyroid hormone is a contributor. I rarely, however, allow weight issues to be my sole indicator to do so, since so many other factors beside thyroid status affect body weight. If a person is fatigued and gaining weight and has a number of other symptoms and some lab data consistent with hypothyroidism, even if only slightly, I'll treat that person with the expectation their weight will benefit. If the person has completely normal labs and the only symptom is weight gain, thyroid pills are unlikely to help.*

CORTISOL

The adrenal glands, located like little hats atop the kidneys, produce several classes of steroid hormones. One is the *glucocorticoid* class, *cortisol* being the major internally produced example, while *hydrocortisone* and *prednisone* are common drugs mimicking the actions of cortisol. I mentioned cortisol in Chapter 2 as having an orexigenic (appetite-stimulating) effect on the hypothalamus of the brain.

Glucocorticoids are necessary for life, and have important roles in metabolism. These steroids function as *stress hormones*: they are released in great quantities in an emergency, such as after a car accident resulting in severe trauma and hemorrhage. Cortisol strengthens the heart, increases blood pressure, mobilizes energy resources. The latter it does by breaking down glucose stores, and proteins and fats, and blocking glucose absorption by all but the most essential of organs—namely, the brain.

Glucocorticoids, in a nutshell, shunt blood, oxygen, and nutrients to the brain to the exclusion of all else. That's a good thing in a crisis, which is always short-lived. In a crisis, the patient either recovers, or dies; either way, the crisis ends.

---

* See my book *The Thyroid Paradox: How to Get the Best Care for Hypothyroidism* (Basic Health Publications, 2007) for a full discussion of how my definition of "normal labs" differs from the typical.

The stress effects of glucocorticoids are bad, however, if we're subjected to them for long periods. This can happen when a tumor produces cortisol, or a stimulator of cortisol release, or in patients taking glucocorticoid drugs for extended periods—prednisone, for example, prescribed to treat asthma or rheumatoid arthritis. The collection of signs and symptoms of too much glucocorticoid is called *Cushing's syndrome.* Among other findings—including high blood pressure, diabetes, weakness, fatigue—*a predominant feature of Cushing's syndrome is obesity.*

Any glucocorticoid medication should be considered the cause of, or contributor to, any unusual weight-management difficulties. Long-term glucocorticoid (often called *corticosteroid*) drug therapy should be avoided if at all possible. If it is needed to treat a serious medical condition, and safe, effective alternatives aren't available, the glucocorticoid dose should be a small as possible, taken as infrequently as possible.

As for a Cushing's-syndrome-related tumor being a possible cause of one's obesity, the chances are remote. Obesity is rampant, Cushing's disease is rare. (Though not strictly correct, I'm using the term *Cushing's disease* to mean any *Cushing's syndrome* not caused by steroid drug therapy, in other words, a tumor-generated Cushing's syndrome.)

It is neither practical nor necessary to screen all obese persons for Cushing's disease, but if questions remain after a physician's thoughtful evaluation, relatively simple tests can rule out adrenal-steroid overproduction. I say *relatively simple* because it isn't as straightforward as, say, glucose testing for diabetes, or thyroid testing for hypothyroidism. Initial screening for Cushing's disease requires a day-long urine collection, or an early-morning blood draw after taking a special pill the night before. And when screening tests come back abnormal, the protocols for determining what, *if anything,* really is wrong, are about the most complicated in modern medicine.

For this reason, it is imperative that laboratory testing for Cushing's disease only be done when true suspicion exists. Such suspicion, in large part, is based upon the appearance of the Cushing's patient, the characteristic distribution of fat over the body. Cushing's syndrome causes so-called *central,* or *centripetal* obesity—fat lost from the arms and legs, and gained in the trunk, neck, and face. Central obesity includes features commonly, and rather rudely, termed a "buffalo hump" and "moon face," and an overall picture one of my mentors called an "apple on a stick." A big belly and thin legs. By contrast "ordinary" obesity is evenly distributed, a person with a big gut also has big thighs, big arms, and so forth. But if the gut is huge and the arms and legs are skinny, especially if other "cushingoid" features are present, an adrenal problem should be sought.

LEPTIN

Adipose tissue (fat) is not simply a passive reservoir for energy storage; it is in fact a complex *endocrine organ*, meaning it makes hormones. A *hormone* is any substance made in one part of the body, secreted directly into the blood, acting elsewhere inside the body. Adipose tissue was recognized as a part of the endocrine system in 1994 with the discovery of *leptin*, produced by the adipocyte (fat cell). Leptin and other adipocyte-secreted substances are now called *adipokines*—nearly 120 of which were known as of 2008.

Leptin is the major communication link between our brain and our fat stores. Leptin is released by fat after we eat and acts on the hypothalamus to suppress chemicals that stimulate feeding (orexigens), and increase others that kill appetite (anorexigens). It also increases energy expenditure, and acts directly on muscle to promote the burning of fat calories. Leptin is a critical regulator of insulin action, individuals genetically lacking leptin having been found to be highly insulin resistant. Leptin also acts on the brain to increase thyroid-hormone production. Leptin levels decline when we fast, resulting in reduced energy expenditure (conservation of fat) mediated partly via lower thyroid levels.

The more adipose tissue people have—that is, the more obese they are—the higher their leptin levels. Why high leptin levels fail to prevent weight gain and reduce eating in obese people has been a mystery. A "leptin resistance syndrome" has been postulated, but an explanation more recently emerging relates to the perverse eating behaviors modern Americans engage in. Leptin is meant to decline when calorie intake is insufficient. Modern "first-world" nutrition, however, is such that calorie intake is almost never insufficient. We in the United States and other affluent societies run high leptin levels all the time, to the point that the mechanism that transports leptin from the blood into the brain is always saturated.

When we eat more than our average, or when we are at an unhealthy weight, more leptin gets produced, but more can't get inside the hypothalamus to the leptin receptor. This might seem like leptin resistance, but in fact there is no resistance; leptin is simply doing all it can for us, all it was ever meant to.

Human leptin is being developed as a drug. Whether it will ever reach market, and if so, how it will be used, remains to be seen. One intriguing possibility under study is the administration of leptin to patients who have lost weight, to help maintain the loss.

WEIGHT-PROMOTING DRUGS

Another of the many ways people differ relates to the drugs prescribed them by their doctors. All drugs can cause side effects and weight gain commonly shows up on those lists. This means part of managing one's unhealthy weight is scrutinizing the medicines you take, and talking to your doctor about whether certain ones can be stopped or changed to alternatives that don't as readily promote obesity.

Diabetes Drugs

There was once upon a time a tragic irony in medicine that the most common drugs used to treat depression—the tricyclic antidepressants—were also amongst the most deadly of pills in the hands of a potentially suicidal person, as some depressed people are. Fortunately, the newer antidepressants are safer.

Along the same lines, it is tragically ironic that many drugs given for diabetes (which as we know promotes and is promoted by obesity) cause significant weight gain. The reason is simple: when blood-sugar control is poor, the kidneys rid the bloodstream of excess sugar by urinating it out. That's why frequent urination is so common a symptom of diabetes. In other words, lots of calories are being flushed down the toilet by the out-of-control diabetic. When insulin shots or certain pills are given to treat diabetes, blood-sugar levels drop because glucose is absorbed into cells all over the body, mostly muscle and fat. In other words, the body is all of a sudden force fed calories that were going down a toilet. Any wonder then that drugs which improve diabetes control often trigger weight gain?

Now, please don't misunderstand: it is critically important to lower high blood-sugar levels regardless, or largely regardless, of any weight gain resulting. High blood sugars wreak crippling havoc on many tissues, including eyes, nerves, kidneys, and the immune system. Fortunately many newer diabetes drugs work in such a manner that weight gain is mitigated. In fact, several antidiabetic drugs—namely metformin and the so called GLP-1 agonists (i.e.,

Byetta, Victoza, and Bydureon)—are being used as weight-loss drugs. In the case of liraglutide (Victoza), FDA approval for obesity treatment is anticipated.

The drugs used for diabetes most notorious for prompting weight gain are as follows:

- All insulins
- Sulfonylureas (glimepiride, glipizide, and glyburide)
- Pioglitazone and rosiglitazone

Antipsychotic/Antidepressant Drugs

The drugs used to treat schizophrenia, bipolar disorder, and extreme anxiety are notorious for causing weight gain and increasing diabetes, hypertension, and hyperlipidemia risk. The biggest offenders amongst the antipsychotics are, in order of descending average weight gain:

- Clozapine (Clozaril)
- Olanzapine (Zyprexa)
- Quetiapine (Seroquel)
- Thioridazine (Mellaril)
- Mesoridazine (Serentil)
- Chlorpromazine (Thorazine)
- Risperidone (Risperdal)
- Haloperidol (Haldol)
- Fluphenazine (Prolixin)

Of note, ziprasidone (Geodon) has consistently proved to be weight neutral, neither increasing nor decreasing weight. Aripiprazole (Abilify) and Molindone (Moban) also carry little to no risk of weight gain.

Already introduced in the above discussion of hypothyroidism and obesity are the antidepressant and "mood-stabilizing" drugs, the latter including lithium, valproic acid (Depakote), carbamazepine (Tegretol), and lamotrigine (Lamictal). Of those, all but lithium are also used in the treatment of epilepsy. Lithium and valproic acid tend to cause significant weight gain, carbamazepine less so, and lamotrigine does not affect weight.

Weight gain is a problem with all tricyclic antidepressants, especially amitriptyline, doxepin, imipramine, and a few others. The newer, more commonly used antidepressants these days, the so-called SSRIs, have variable effects on weight which may even include an initial weight loss early in treatment, but eventual weight gain which can be very persistent. The worst offender is paroxetine (Paxil), compared to which sertraline (Zoloft) and especially fluoxetine (Prozac) are associated with lesser to no weight gain. There is also a diverse group of drugs known as atypical antidepressants, among which, weight problems are common and substantial with mirtazapine (Remeron), while nefazodone (Serzone) is weight neutral and bupropion (Wellbutrin) may even produce a modest weight loss, to the extent that bupropion may have some utility as an anti-obesity drug.

Other Weight-Promoting Drugs

Additional drugs for the person with a weight problem to be wary of include, as already mentioned, glucocorticoids, like prednisone, progestational sex steroids like Prometrium, antihistamines, beta blockers such as metoprolol (but not carvedilol), and alpha blockers such as doxazosin.

CONCLUSION

If you are eating "exactly" the same, exerting "exactly" the same, day in and day out, as your friend or spouse and they are losing weight and you aren't, *don't* decide something is wrong with you and give up, or be frustrated or mystified. It just means you're different and you, unfortunately, must work harder, or at least differently to achieve the same result. Some of the diversity accounting for different responses to weight-loss efforts are unmodifiable—such as one's sex or genetic structure. Other diversity might be modifiable, such as a disease like hypothyroidism, or very rarely (let me emphasize that) tumor-associated Cushing's syndrome, or the use of certain prescriptions drugs. In particular, if you are at an unhealthy weight and can't seem to readily reduce, *pay close attention to any prescription drugs you are taking, do your own research, and discuss them with your doctor.* It would be irresponsible and potentially risky to stop anything on your own, but in consultation with your doctor it might be possible to stop or substitute for a drug that is contributing to your weight problem. Particular drug classes to pay attention to are those used to treat diabetes and mental-health disorders, including depression. Also steroids and beta blockers.

9

ENVIRONMENTAL VARIABLES

The last two chapters detailed gender-specific, genetic, pathologic, and pharmacologic factors that make one person different from another, altering their tendencies toward obesity, and response to weight-loss efforts. I debated where to include the next two factors, deciding to give them their own chapter, since they are so unique, and under recognized, and potentially critical.

Let me just say, the smartest people specializing in obesity medicine are only now beginning to get a handle on the multitude of factors contributing to the obesity epidemic on a global scale, as well as the weight-management concerns of any given patient. And it has recently become apparent to me that the complexity of obesity, and of what needs to be done to manage it, far exceeds the common understanding of the average layperson, and for that matter, the average physician. I enter the remainder of this chapter into evidence, supporting that contention.

BISPHENOL A

When I read a February 2013 commentary by two Melbourne, Australia diabetologists in the *Journal of Clinical Endocrinology and Metabolism*—titled (and what a title!): "Bisphenol A and Diabetes, Insulin Resistance, Cardiovascular Disease and Obesity: Controversy in a (Plastic) Cup?"—it occurred to me how bizarrely ironic it would be if what we eat and drink were less important to the epidemic of obesity than the container it was packaged in and consumed from.

Bisphenol A (BPA) is a ubiquitous environmental chemical. It is a primary component of polycarbonate, a hard, clear plastic used to make a host of consumer products, including CDs and DVDs! BPA is a basic ingredient in the epoxy resins that line canned foods and drinks. The largest source of human BPA ingestion is from food packaging, but BPA has also been detected in dust and air particles, dental sealants, and water. And in the past five years, human epidemiological studies have provided rapidly mounting evidence linking BPA to obesity, diabetes and cardiovascular disease. As far back as 2007, I noted a report that BPA might interfere with thyroid hormone action, which might be expected to promote obesity, in my book *The Thyroid Paradox*. A 2008 study showed that BPA inhibits adiponectin, a key beneficial regulator of insulin action and tissue inflammation. To make matters worse, it is now suspected that previous FDA and EPA estimates of human exposure to BPA were low.

BPA may be the tip of the iceberg. It is the environmental endocrine-disruptor toxicant that we know about, that is getting all the attention, but it is likely to be one of many common chemical exposures—related to electronic insulation, plasticizers, and pesticides, as examples—associated with chronic disease.

How do we at least avoid BPA?

I'm not sure that we do, short of a government ban, though the robust studies needed to drive such an action against the powerful petrochemical industry are lacking, and are expensive and difficult to do. If you know anything about BPA at all you know that the manufacturers of baby bottles and sports-water bottles have voluntarily eliminated it, and you know that that recycling code #7 is best avoided. However, as I said above, BPA is not limited to baby and sports-water bottles, nor even to products that have that recycling number on them. Even so, it is widely acknowledged that those recycling numbers are highly inaccurate, that it is virtually impossible for the ordinary consumer to really know what's in their plastic product, and that in some cases the manufacturers don't even fully know the heritage of the plastic stock they use.

I won't claim I've eliminated BPA from my life. There does come a time when you have to live in the real world, play the poker hand you're dealt, as it were. That said, I make a point of buying products in glass rather than plastic, when that alternative reasonably presents itself. An example is olive oil: grocery-store displays present me with numerous alternatives, some in plastic bottles, some in glass, and I automatically eliminate the ones in plastic from consideration.

So, let's say you *are* doing everything "right."

Maybe you're just overweight from the lining of your canned goods and the BPA leeching into the atmosphere from your CD collection.

I exaggerate—slightly—but these factors might well be a contributor to your concerns.

GUT MICROBIOTA

I mentioned the role bacteria living in our digestive tracts have in the metabolism of ingested food back in Chapter 2. I also mentioned these bacteria may be involved in determining one's propensity to develop of obesity. This is part of a fascinating recent area of research—I see a new scientific report or even newspaper article about this almost daily—suggesting that in some sense, obesity may well be an infectious disease. There is a common type of virus, for example, called Ad-36, that has been shown to cause weight gain in chickens and mice, and there is human data to suggest that Ad-36 exposure is associated with higher BMI and body-fat percentage.

Most of this compelling research, though, involves bacteria residing in the GI tract. It is becoming clear that one's gut-microbial profile (the specific species of bacteria comprising the gut microbiota of a given person) has an effect on body weight. It may be that the greater the variety of bacteria one carries, the healthier one's weight. One of the effects of Roux-en-Y gastric bypass (RYGB), a common type of bariatric surgery (surgery to treat obesity), is to change the gut microbiota. If you transfer bacteria harvested from the intestines of a mouse who has undergone RYGB into a germ-free mouse, the second mouse loses weight. If you do the same experiment, but harvest the gut microbiota of a mouse that did not get a RYGB, and transfer that into a germ-free mouse, the second mouse gains weight.

You can do the same without surgery—transferring the gut microbiota of a lean mouse to another mouse induces leanness in the second mouse, while transferring from an obese mouse leads to obesity in the second mouse. Besides surgery, an number of interventions can reshape the gut microbiota, either increasing or decreasing body weight and body fat. Pregnancy, vitamin D, and changes in diet, for example, all effect changes in the intestinal bacteria profile, that influence weight, either up or down. A 2013 paper in *Endocrine Practice* reports that vitamin D supplementation and foods rich in vitamin D (certain fishes, for example), as well as prebiotics improve glucose levels in T2DM and prediabetes, through modification of the gut microbiota. *Prebiotics* are nondigestible foods that reach the large intestine and can be fermented by the bacteria residing there. These include artichokes, onion, garlic, barley, rye and wheat bran, and asparagus.

Obviously antibiotic drugs affect the gut microbiota. We can thus add antibiotics to our list of weight-promoting drugs from the last chapter. And it is not any one antibiotic either. It's all of them. For practical proof of this look no further than the common practice of low-dose antibiotic use in farming to promote the growth of animals. Farmers also of course medicate their stock with antibiotics to prevent the spread of infectious diseases amongst the animals. Thus, to the extent these drugs, used for various purposes in the food-production chain, survive in the tissues of slaughtered animals, and in harvested eggs, there is the potential for much unintended human antibiotic ingestion, further promoting patient-care-relevant antibiotic resistance (a public-health issue beyond the scope of this book) and obesity.

In other words, you don't even have to take a penicillin prescription for strep throat, or the like, to be exposed to obesity-promoting antibiotics. (The same can be said, by the way, of steroids used in livestock production).

How do gut bacteria affect energy balance?

Part of the answer is remarkably simple. Bacteria have to eat too. They metabolize nutrients for their own energy needs. And lest you think this is insignificant, remember, there are ten fold more bacterial cells in and on a human body than there are human cells. Gut microbes also produce or alter various signals affecting fatty acid metabolism and adipose-tissue growth, and certain bacteria harbor toxins that trigger inflammation, which might, for example, worsen insulin resistance. If some intervention promotes the growth of good bacteria, which then compete with the bad bacteria for resources, the human host may benefit.

The gut-microbiota/obesity connection is generating a lot of excitement, though more work is needed to figure out how to use this information. We might get to the point where a specific obesity-resistant collection of bacteria could be inoculated directly into one's intestinal tract, or could be introduced through ingestion of the right *probiotic* (therapeutic preparations of microorganisms administered in oral form). Don't get overeager though and run to your favorite health-food store for the latest bestselling probiotic. The chance you'll hit on the right bacterial concoction is remote, and it is questionable, in any case, how effective swallowed bacteria are at altering meaningfully, sustainedly, the existing gut microbiota. Perhaps, one day, obesity therapy might involve high-doses of broad-spectrum antibiotics to wipe out an existing unfavorable gut flora, followed by introduction of a new, more weight-friendly collection of bacteria. That's pure speculation on my part, and we certainly aren't there yet.

For now, my suggestion is vitamin D—especially if you are deficient—and a plant-based, high-fiber diet to promote intestinal bacterial activity. It may well be, the "gassier" you are, the healthier you are. Or as my step-father in law famously said: "A fartin' horse is a workin' horse."

10

EAT & DRINK LESS—A LOT LESS

For a weight-loss guide to have a chapter titled as this one may seem elementary—off-putting, even, to those sincerely believing they are overweight or obese in spite of an absolutely appropriate diet. I truly wish I had a dime for every patient who has said to me, "I'm eating what I'm supposed to," or "I have a healthy diet," or the like, as if that mattered.

(I know, I keep harping on that but I truly believe stubborn adherence to what we think, for whatever reason, to be healthy, rather than thinking outside the box, trying different diets, is one of the major blockades to successful obesity management.)

It is perfectly possible to be eating what might generally be considered a "healthy" diet, and still gain weight or fail to lose weight. The causes of obesity are many and diverse. There is no one "healthy diet." There is no "supposed to" when it comes to weight management. Energy balance in the body is complex and regulated. There is more to it that just calorie intake. It is physiologically normal for the human body to look at a weight loss resulting from a conscientious decrease in food intake, and turn right around and deliberately cut basal metabolism for the purpose of bringing the weight back up to the brain's set point. Reducing calorie intake alone may not result in sustained weight loss. A combination of things needs to be tried. Different things need to be tried. Something drastic needs to change in order to "shock" the body into lowering that set point, otherwise the body will always bring you back home to that weight you're trying to get away from. There is more to losing weight than just eating fewer calories.

But: *eating fewer calories is nevertheless critical.*

It is a first step or part of a first step. For example, eating different types of foods might be as important as cutting calories, but calories must be cut. In the end we must eat fewer calories than we burn off, and however complicated achieving that balance might be, however strongly the body might be holding down the wrong side of the teeter-totter, eating less is always going to help, even it's just a nudge in the right direction. Because, always remember, and never forget...

It is physically impossible to gain fat that was not first swallowed as some form of food or beverage. This chapter is about food and beverages, and being more responsible with them. They may not be the whole story, but they are the part of the story we're dealing with now.

So, forget what and how much you think you *should* eat and drink. *What should work* is medically irrelevant. *What proves to work* is all that matters. Those most likely to be successful managing weight—same for diabetes, by the way—are those who can stop being frustrated over the failure of what they are doing, and try something totally new and different. We must dispense with the notion that there is any single "correct" diet. We've seen how weight outcomes differ depending on gender, genetic factors, medical history, habitual activity levels. Environment plays a role too: the same person can eat more without gaining weight at the South Pole than in sunny Florida, owing to greater body-heat production in frigid environments.

Put simply:

Everything is relative.

We should not be eating foods laced with hemlock, or only trans fats, or only simple sugars, but beyond avoiding the poisonous or recklessly unbalanced, there is a wide range of appropriate nutrition. The trick is finding the "right" diet for the individual in question. And we need a strategy for accomplishing that.

FOODS

Most of us eat more than we should. Some get away with it better than others, but most modern Americans consume more calories than their bodies need, as attested to by the "maxed-out" leptin discussion of Chapter 8. And in an earlier chapter, I cited the interesting fact that, according to Harvard's Dr. Kaplan, all mammals, including humans, do consume far more calories than are needed in an average day, and their bodies routinely burn off that excess. Supported by that observation, I think few modern

Americans have the foggiest notion how little food we can get away with and still be healthy and happy. We have a distorted notion of what healthy eating looks like, born out of the relative affluence of even the poorest of us, compared to third-world populations, and earlier generations of Americans.

Much of what we eat is a want, not a need, but we don't recognize *want* versus *need* because most of us have lived our entire lives able to obtain pretty much anything we want to eat, in pretty much any quantity. Most of us can buy from a grocery store, or order in a restaurant of some caliber, almost any variety of food, in relatively large serving sizes. Case in point, the all-you-can-eat Chinese buffet. Is there an American city or town of any size that doesn't have one?

We are fortunate to live in a society of plenty and variety, but we also suffer for it. We are immersed in *super-sizing, all you can eat, you can't leave the table till you've cleaned your plate, value for the money,* and so forth. I'm not saying most people don't know that eating a literal mound of food at the Chinese buffet, then going back for seconds—it happens!—is inconsistent with effective weight loss. However, I do think most Americans fail to limit themselves, and fail to recognize many examples of overeating. In Japan, a standard sushi portion is one ounce of fish; in the United States, two ounces. Walk down the candy aisle at your local convenience store. Some of those Snickers bars are huge compared to when I was a kid, and I have to look pretty hard to find a peanut-butter cup in just a two-pack. On the top shelf they always have the four-pack, or the extra big Reese's cup. Obesity-medicine experts call this *portion distortion.*

So, real weight-loss strategy number one:

Eat less.

What's the worst that can happen? You might get hungry. So what? What we call hunger, for the most part, is not third-world hunger that kills people. Yet, that seems a revelation to some I talk to—that hunger pangs, a growling stomach, are not life and death. They may be very hard to ignore, but they are not life and death.

Leave some space on your plate.

Get what you want, within reason, but no seconds.

Even if you aren't a vegetarian, have a vegetarian day now and then.

If you want a food you know to be unhealthy or high-calorie, take a small portion, one or two bites.

Two bread slices per sandwich? Cut one into halves and fold the same amount of meat between them. Or, if a sandwich has been prepared for you, remove one piece of bread and fold everything into the remaining piece.

Take one biscuit or roll, never two.

Better yet, tear one in half.

My wife's step-mother makes these great cookies for Christmas. I break one in half and leave the rest. The family gripes about those "cookie stumps" left behind, but even if my willpower fails and I go back for the other half, I still end up eating less, because if I ate the whole cookie to begin with, I still might want another.

They're Claire Verdura's Chootchy-dots after all!

We eat food in units, tending to finish whatever is in front of us. In this regard, visual cues override appetite-driven ones. If the food package is large, we eat it all—buy smaller packages, serve smaller portions. Cutting food, such as meat, into smaller pieces creates the appearance of more food and can fool the brain into getting full faster. Whatever you do, don't trust serving sizes in restaurants and packaged foods, nor can you blindly trust your own appetite. In an experiment known as the "bottomless bowl" study in 2003, subjects were told to eat soup until they were full. Half ate from a normal bowl and half, unbeknownst to them, from a bowl rigged to inconspicuously refill itself!

The refilling-bowl group ate 73 percent more soup!

Three meals every day?

Eat a small snack for supper instead of making it the biggest meal like most do.

At the Chinese buffet: make a rule, a code to live by (live *better* by!). Never, ever go back for seconds. Get whatever you want, first time through, but don't go back.

Lastly, do not ever let anybody, I don't care who—mother, mother-in-law, whoever—shame you into eating more. If you want it, that's one thing. That's a different challenge. If somebody else thinks you should have it, say no and politely explain—but do not give in.

BEVERAGES TOO

Drink is an important source of excess calories: supremely important because liquids don't send the same fullness signals that solid food does. Since they don't suppress food intake much, beverage calories are mostly "add-on" calories. And liquids are rapidly absorbed, requiring little if any digestion, and are often heavily sweetened, often unnaturally.

Now, regardless of whether the intestinal absorption rate and macronutrient composition (fats vs. carbs vs. proteins) of a particular bunch of calories matter with respect to its ultimate impact on BMI—the traditional view would be that they don't, which I disagree with—but regardless, I mention here the often-sugary composition of and ease of absorption of liquids (and for that matter, ease of ingestion—nobody ever chugalugged a cheeseburger!), mainly for their tendency to aggravate high blood sugars in the diabetic or prediabetic.*

And with respect to diabetes risk it clearly does matter whether calories come from fat, or carbohydrates, or protein. In data pooled from 175 different countries, an increase in calorie intake of 150 calories per person per day slightly increased the prevalence of diabetes by 0.1 percent. But, if that 150-calorie increase was sugar, roughly equivalent to adding a can of real soda per day, the diabetes rate increased 1.1 percent. An 11-fold difference. "Let me repeat," Dr. Robert H. Lustig of the University of California at San Francisco wrote, "the total calories did not count." All that mattered was sugar calories, meaning sweet beverages are uniquely diabetogenic. The New York City Health Commissioner, commenting on that city's efforts to ban sales of large sugary drinks, added: "This is the largest single driver of the obesity epidemic...It is the largest source of added sugars to our diet."

Fluid intake is good and necessary, especially in hot climates, especially after physical exertion and sweating, especially in the elderly, who have a lower percentage of body water to start with. But it needs to mostly be water, which is calorie free and will not contribute to obesity or diabetes.†

Praise for Water

Our bodies are mostly water, the percentage varying, but around 60 percent. In severe obesity, interestingly, water might account for as little as 45 percent of body weight, since fat tends to displace, rather than hold onto water.

Drinking water, pure water, replenishes what we are, the medium

---

* *Prediabetes* is a condition of "borderline" high blood sugars that don't yet meet the criteria for diabetes, but which indicate a high risk of future diabetes.

† Notice, I didn't say *weight*; retained water does contribute to weight, but not to excess fat, which is the only weight this book is concerned with.

in which all the chemistry that runs our physiology takes place. To drink pure water is the most natural way to maintain and replenish our body fluids: "natural" being a watchword frequently used by those concerned with health, which may or may not be of medical significance, but it's a word that gets hyped a lot, and carries weight with the public. So I urge you to hydrate "naturally" with water. Most of us don't need the salts in the sports drinks—and those who do, don't need them to the exclusion of water, only to augment water's benefits.

Yet I've often had patients tell me:

"I don't like water."

"I can't stand the taste of it."

"I can't make myself drink it."

To them, I say: water is what God and/or Mother Nature intended for us to drink and anything else is mucking up the works. You may not like the taste of pipes in tap water; in fact, my wife won't drink tap water. We get filtered water out of a spigot in the refrigerator and have a water-filtering pitcher. She drinks that. You can try bottled and jug waters. I'm urging water consumption as a way of avoiding the additives to water that are in every other beverage. Additives like sugar (lots of sugar, including high-fructose corn syrup), caffeine, fat (in milk and cream), and of course alcohol. And all those additives, except for caffeine, add up to calories, calories, calories.

In a recent opinion piece in *Internal Medicine News*, Dr. Jon Ebbert, a Mayo Clinic professor of medicine, stated: "Drinking water in lieu of sugar-sweetened beverages has been shown to reduce total energy intake, increase the feeling of fullness, reduce the perception of hunger, and increase energy expenditure."

Sounds to me like water does everything one would want a "diet drink" to do, but which, as we will see, I'm not convinced those beverage products labeling themselves "diet" actually, in fact, do.

Soda

Mass-produced carbonated beverages are everywhere: grocery stores, vending machines, gas stations, convenience marts in even our poorest neighborhoods. They come in 12- and 16-ounce cans, 20-ounce bottles, insane 32-ounce Big Gulp fountain drink cups. I'll give the two- and three-liter bottles a pass, as intended for consumption by a household, or a gathering; however, I recall a patient whose diabetes we couldn't get under control—and, oh by the way, she was drinking two or three of those big bottles of Pepsi a day! Yes, people do these things!

When I was a kid Cokes came in 6.5-ounce and Mountain Dew in 12-ounce bottles. Sweetened with cane sugar, not high-fructose corn syrup. What was a tasty, basically safe (if not healthy) treat in small quantities, has morphed into slow poison consumed in large volumes by many people around the clock. Given that this chapter is about cutting calories, I'll grant that substituting diet sodas for real sodas should be a way of doing that. However, they are not a straight-up safe alternative to water. It is not even clear that they help people lose weight (see Chapter 14). For example, Dr. Ebbert, the Mayo Clinic water proponent, believes low-calorie and no-calorie sweeteners, may "'prime' consumers for sweetness—leading to increased caloric consumption with the next meal."

Another potential problem with the average soda, even diet soda: they usually contain caffeine, stimulating the central nervous system, providing positive reinforcement, promoting further consumption of the same beverage.

Milk

Most of us would agree that sugary sodas, especially in large volumes, are not healthy. What about other liquids that are, by reputation, healthier? Milk, for example. For those people not allergic, or intestinally intolerant, milk can be a nutritious drink, in moderation. Its calcium is important, as is the Vitamin D milk products are often fortified with. It would be hard—not to mention, unadvisable—to drink enough milk to adequately supply those nutrients, but, every little bit helps. Milk does contain sugar and protein, as well as fat, except for skim (fat-free) milk. These components combine to make it a relatively high-calorie beverage (eight ounces of whole milk contains 146 calories, more than 12-ounces of regular Coke), meaning it could adversely affect BMI, diabetes, and hyperlipidemia. And both whole and skim milk contain the same amount of lactose (milk sugar), which ends up being, ounce for ounce, about half the sugar regular Coke contains. If you're a milk drinker, organic products might be healthier than conventionally produced one, less likely to be contaminated by pesticides, hormones, and antibiotics dairy cattle might be exposed to.

In small quantities cow's milk is an excellent beverage, but it contains too much other stuff to recommend it as a vehicle for hydration. People with diabetes or hyperlipidemia should stick with skim milk, but don't forget the sugar content, which is as great as whole milk. And remember, anyone following a nutritional lifestyle with the goal of losing weight and/or controlling diabetes, will almost always be better off with zero-calorie/zero-carb water.

Juice

Ah, juice—that stuff even people focused on, nay, obsessed with healthy eating and drinking often mistakenly believe to be just peachy for them (pun intended), a freebie, they can quaff with relish. My Upstate New York mother-in-law spends winters in Florida and called me once worried her new cholesterol medicine meant she couldn't drink her huge glasses of cold grapefruit juice she so loved. I told her I thought she was crazy to drink down that much sugar regardless of her drug-interaction concern, and regardless of the fact it was "juice" she was drinking.

Just the other day I had one of those patients who couldn't lose weight despite doing everything "right." I asked what she was doing that she considered "right" and her first answer was "juicing." I asked whether she had a family history of diabetes and she said everybody in her family had diabetes. Question answered. What she was doing wrong, or at least one thing she was doing wrong, was juicing! She was genetically programmed to react badly to sugar (the diabetes history) and she was pulverizing with eager enthusiasm lots of sugar-laden fruit down to a rapidly absorbable liquid form.

We need to think, and evaluate, not just accept labels, and long-held assumptions at face value, assumptions like "juice is good," and "fat is bad."

What is *juice*?

Presumably we mean fruit juice, the liquid resulting from crushing, squeezing, blending, or otherwise macerating the edible sweet-pulp-containing reproductive body of a seed plant. In other words, juice is processed; the more processed a food is, the less "natural" it is, and potentially the less healthy.

Better perhaps to just eat the fruit.

If a given juice product was really made from the fruit it's purported to be, processed by methods preserving a reasonable amount of the vitamins, minerals, other nutrients contained in the original fruit, especially if some vestige of the original remains, like pulp in orange juice, then that juice product is healthier than soda.

But juices have calories.

They are not freebies when it comes to weight.

The main thing about juice is, read the label, know exactly what's in that bottle before you drink it. Not uncommonly apple juice is artificially flavored to mimic something else, pomegranate juice, or whatever. Worse yet, some beverage products look like, and are packaged like, might even be shelved alongside real juices, yet their main ingredient is high-fructose corn syrup, in which case the product is hardly better than soda. The claim "100% natural" is reassuring, but I still urge reading the fine print.

Drunk in moderation, truly all-natural juices are a better choice than soda. Just as with milk, though, don't drink juices in large quantities.

Save the chugging for water.

Coffee

Coffee has been popular the world over for centuries, and remains so, evidenced by the plethora of Starbucks and Seattle's Bests and the like. Coffee has had ups and downs with respect to medicine's take on it. Certainly caffeine intake has been a perennial concern related to heart disease and high blood pressure, and there was a scare some years back about coffee and pancreatic cancer. The cancer worry never bore out. At this time the pendulum is swinging in favor of coffee as a relatively healthful drink. A 2006 report in *Diabetes Care* linked coffee consumption to a 60 percent lower risk of type 2 diabetes. A 2009 paper in the same journal showed no increased risk of cardiovascular disease or death in diabetic men drinking four or more cups of coffee per day. A 2012 *New England Journal of Medicine* piece reported from a large well-designed study that increasing coffee consumption correlated with lower death rates overall, and due to specific diseases. For what it's worth, the great French writer and philosopher Voltaire, who died in 1778 at the age of 83, when normal life expectancy was probably half that, is said to have drunk between fifty and seventy cups of coffee per day!

A condition related to obesity we have not spoken of before, but will meet again, is *nonalcoholic fatty liver*, which can progress to the more serious chronic liver disease *nonalcoholic steatohepatitis*, or NASH, which further progresses to cirrhosis a quarter of the time. NASH kills 40 percent of sufferers over ten years. If we look at patients with *cirrhosis*—end-stage, often-fatal congestion and failure of the liver—when there is no other apparent cause, such as alcoholism or infection, 74 percent are obese or have diabetes. Weight loss has been shown to improve NASH, and prevent cirrhosis, which I why we're talking about the liver in a weight-loss book. Coffee also can prevent or improve NASH, which is why I bring it up here.

In fact, consuming two cups of coffee per day reduces hospitalizations and mortality from chronic liver disease by more than half.

Why is coffee protective against death, liver and heart disease, and diabetes?

No one knows.

But an effect of caffeine on metabolic rate, body-heat generation, and reduced obesity rates, has been seen in some studies. Other researchers have focused on compounds in coffee beans other than caffeine, since decaffeinated coffees also benefit glucose metabolism. Coffee drinkers have higher adiponectin levels, a substance that reduces insulin resistance and inflammation. It is likely that caffeine in combination with these other compounds is responsible for coffee's benefits. I also believe there to be a simpler benefit:

I believe a person who drinks a lot of coffee, is less likely to drink excessive amounts of sugary sodas. Either because they're spending all their time drinking coffee, or because coffee-drinking serves the same quick-pick-me-up function. That is, heavy coffee consumption and heavy soda consumption might be largely mutual exclusive.

One positive attribute of coffee per se is that it contains no calories. In many ways it's "water with benefits." It has no calories but does have taste, and the other benefits detailed above.

What's the down side?

None, if you drink your coffee black.

If you load it full of sugar and cream, worse yet, flavored syrups, you are negating some, perhaps most, even all, of the benefit. The jury is still out on those little blue, yellow, and pink packets of artificial sweeteners—again, more on that later.

My advice…

Drink coffee black.

And drink a lot of it.

I'm a big fan of coffee. Personally and professionally. For the record, I drink no more than one real 12-ounce soda per day, and the rest of the day, till the cocktail hour anyway, I drink water and black unsweetened coffee.

Period.

11

CREATURES OF HABIT

This chapter continues the eat- (and drink-) less theme of the last chapter, which in part introduced some suggested behaviors for fostering reduced food consumption, in particular, smaller portion sizes. We branched off into a discussion of various types of liquid consumption, a deceptively dangerous source of add-on calories, especially sugar calories. At this point I want to return to what experts call *behavioral treatment of obesity*—the notion that new eating and activity habits can be learned in the same manner as a sport or musical instrument.

Changing habits requires *positive reinforcement*, some perceived benefit that follows the altered behavior, encouraging a repeating of that behavior. I think attitude is important—a positive attitude, that anticipates, searches for, the slightest good result from a reduced consumption of calories. A healthier BMI, perhaps better diabetes control, are what we're ultimately seeking, but those things come slowly, too slowly to be immediately useful reinforcers.

The person with the positive attitude needs to seek, latch onto earlier, subtler benefits—things good in themselves, making them better reinforcers, but which are really just indicators that we're getting there. In medicine, we call these *surrogate markers*.

A lower LDL cholesterol is a surrogate marker for reduced heart-disease risk. The goal of treatment isn't so much cholesterol reduction—LDL, after all, doesn't make people feel bad—the goal is to live longer, not having had a heart attack or stroke along the way. The LDL test, if it's improving, is early positive reinforcement that keep us eating right and taking our statin drugs, when many years must elapse before we can look back with satisfaction and say, wow, no heart attack, and I'm still alive and breathing.

ACCENTUATE THE POSITIVE

What are some surrogate markers heralding a future lower BMI, that might reinforce eating less? How about post-meal discomfort—fullness in the abdomen, a tightening of the belt, sluggishness and fatigue. Eat less and you won't have all that. It will feel good and you'll remember that good feeling next time you eat. Fullness also promotes acid reflux, and makes it harder to sleep. Focus on these positives and you'll want to eat less, and it won't be such a struggle.

SLOW IT DOWN

Another habit that leads to eating less is eating slowly. When we eat slowly we allow time for hormonal signals from the gut (like GLP-1, cholecystokinin, pancreatic polypeptide) to tell the brain we are full, weakening the appetite we started our meal with. It takes around twenty minutes for these signals to kick in. Take the same plate of food: gorge it down in ten minutes, you'll eat the whole plate; take thirty minutes, you'll feel full toward the end, and maybe skip a few forkfuls.

Something that helps us eat more slowly, I think, is elevating the quality and flavor of the foods we eat. This makes us want to savor them, keep them on the tongue longer, rather than slamming them down because we're hungry and that's all we care about.

Food quality will be the focus of the next chapter.

A female friend I was having lunch with the other day told me she knew someone who said a blessing between each bite of food, and was losing weight as a result. It occurred to me what she was really doing was slowing her eating. The blessing was a technique for doing that that worked for her. A great example of how different things work for different people: keep trying until you find what works for you. Speaking of eating slow, when I eat oriental food I use those chopsticks they give you. I can't get too big a bite from my plate to my mouth between two chopsticks, and that's good. Makes me eat slower. I don't know if it's true or not that oriental ethnicity is associated with lower obesity rates, but that's the stereotype.

Is the lowly chopstick responsible?

MEAL STRUCTURE/PLANNING

We might eat less if we rethink our ingrained assumptions regarding the role and composition of each of the three traditional meals:

- Breakfast
- Lunch
- Dinner

I've heard advice about only eating when you're hungry. That might work for some, but to me that plan seems too freewheeling, and ultimately self-defeating. I think some structure, timetable, habit is needed for long-term success. I don't trust leaving food consumption to be guided by hunger. Hunger is very subjective, and if you go till you're really hungry, till you're famished, you'll eat more than you would have if you were sticking to a plan, eating on a schedule. In fact, there is data showing that more structure regarding meals is associated with greater weight loss—"structure" referring to prefabricated meals and meal-replacement products, such as those provided through commercial weight-loss concerns like Nutrisystem. That's one way to achieve structure, but not the only way. You can do it on your own, cheaper, by establishing regular habits, and including meal plans into those habits.

I suggest eating at least three meals on a roughly stable schedule every day. My comments assume a typical daytime nine-to-five-ish work or school schedule, but can be modified to other routines. If you snack in between meals, establish regular habits for that too. Nothing should be a surprise to you or your body. At the very least, if it's working you'll know what to stick with, and if it's not you'll have an easier time figuring out what to change.

It's fairly common in our society to eat little if any breakfast, a fairly small, perhaps rushed lunch, and a huge belt-bursting supper at the end of the day. If you have that big evening meal at home, with your family around the table, talking, sharing news of each other's lives, that's an important positively reinforcing activity. It is not however healthy, least of all if you need to lose weight.

Everyone should eat breakfast.

In fact, there is a widely held presumption in obesity medicine (current data neither proves nor disproves it definitively) that *eating breakfast is a nearly universal characteristic of people who lose weight and keep it off.* I think we should eat fairly big breakfasts, fairly balanced for carbohydrates, proteins, and fats. They'll satisfy you through the morning and you'll be less likely to feel a need to snack before lunch. Similarly I encourage a fairly substantial lunch that will satisfy through the afternoon. This advice may seem to contradict the eat-less theme, so let me explain.

If you are trying to lose weight and/or control diabetes or high cholesterol, you need to look at your portions, and reduce them, so that total calorie intake over the day is cut. When I talk about eating a substantial breakfast and lunch, I'm speaking in relative terms. Whatever that reduced daily calorie intake is, should be apportioned over the three meals, but that apportionment doesn't have to be even. In fact, we've already agreed the typical American meal schedule is not even, but skewed toward a large supper. I'm saying to shift that skew earlier in the day. The larger meals should fuel and sustain you through busy, active times, and in the evening, when you're going to be relaxing, watching TV, talking, reading, going to bed, eat very little. Just a snack—cheese, grapes, slice of deli meat— or a small meal like a soup or salad. I like a little something at bedtime. I eat one palm full of bran cereal.

No milk.

Dry cereal.

My proposal to eat more calories earlier in the day is supported by a 2013 paper in the *International Journal of Obesity*, looking at 420 overweight or obese people in Spain. Now, in Spain, the traditional largest meal (in the study, 40% of total calories) is lunch. This research compared those who ate lunch before three p.m. and those who ate lunch after three p.m. The late eaters lost weight more slowly and "lost significantly less weight than early eaters," according to Harvard neuroscientist Frank Scheer.

Say your current calorie intake is 2000 per day and you've decided to cut that to 1500. I'm not a fan, remember, of calorie counting—I eyeball portion sizes, assess the outcome, then readjust accordingly—I'm just using calorie counts here for illustration. I might divide that 1500 calories into 600 each at breakfast and lunch, and 300 at supper. Now, those might sound like low calorie intakes and, again, I'm just tossing numbers around as examples. I'm not writing a nutritional prescription for anybody. But a significant calorie reduction shifts your metabolism from an energy-storage program—bad—to an energy-mobilization program—good. Mobilization of fat stores in the skin and abdomen, movement of dangerous fatty infiltrations out of internal organs, such as the liver and pancreas. This new energy-mobilization physiology (which you are going to maintain, because, remember, no "diets" here, only "lifestyles") will include lower insulin levels, smoother blood sugar fluctuations, and better diabetes control.

Research dating back to 1935 shows calorie-restricted rats have extended life spans. A 2009 paper in *Science* reported a 60 percent greater survival rate over a twenty-year period in a group of rhesus monkeys fed 30 percent fewer calories than a control group of monkeys allowed to eat whatever they wanted. The calorie-restricted monkeys had less diabetes, cancer, cardiovascular disease, and age-related brain shrinkage. It is not always accurate to extrapolate animal data to humans, but in this case it makes sense, knowing everything else we know, that a sustained lower-calorie diet—sufficient and supplemented enough to avoid malnutrition—might well stave off death and disease.

I am not suggesting starvation, nor wholesale skipping of meals as a weight-control method. I'm suggesting low but regular calorie intake to keep you satisfied and the metabolic engine running, in an energy-burning, rather than energy-storing state. Starvation is counter-productive. Starvation would be a low, irregular energy intake, and would, for example, stop conversion of thyroxine (T4), the major thyroid hormone, to its active metabolite, triiodothyronine (T3). Lower T3 levels result in a lower metabolism, representing the body's effort to conserve resources in the face of what, for all it knows, might be the next Irish potato famine—the exact opposite of what you want if you want to lose weight.

Two Versus Six?

At the annual scientific sessions of the American Diabetes Association in 2013, Dr. Hana Kahleová, a diabetologist from Prague, Czech Republic, presented research comparing a two-meals-per-day diet (a hearty breakfast and lunch, the latter not later than four p.m.) with a six-meals-per-day diet in fifty-four T2DM patients. Six meals per day is a commonly recommended diabetes meal plan. Both diets provided the same restricted energy intake of 500 calories per day, and the same percentages of fats, carbohydrates, and protein.

The two-meal diet resulted in 50 percent greater BMI reduction after twelve weeks, as well as improvements in blood sugars, liver fat content, and insulin resistance. Dr. Kahleová stated that her research "supported the ancient proverb: Eat breakfast like a king, lunch like a prince, and dinner like a pauper."

12

QUALITY NOT QUANTITY

My mother preached this chapter's title aphorism. She would pay $5 for one really good doohickey—much to my late, budget-minded father's exasperation—rather than the same on two half-good doohickeys. She was the opposite of a *value* shopper, someone looking to buy more for less. I won't judge which is the better consumer strategy. The answer no doubt depends on the individual and his or her socioeconomic status, and what function the doohickey serves. If we're talking mountain-climbing gear, and some gizmo is going to be holding me swaying a thousand feet above some rocky chasm, I'm probably going to pony up more bucks for the best quality gizmo they make. If we're talking cereal bowls, I might just as soon buy a plastic one than a Wedgwood china one, and put the savings toward better mountain-climbing gear.

My wife, paying attention to the bathroom scale, thinks of calories in terms of their cost with respect to their effect on her weight, and she has a quality-versus-quantity rule of thumb about eating. To explain, I'll turn to another adage: *A moment on the lips, a lifetime on the hips.* The lifetime on the hips (or abdomen, or infiltrating the liver) is, to my wife's thinking, the *cost* of that moment on the lips. Applying quality-not-quantity to that equation, she won't pay the price unless the moment on the lips is really, really good—top quality.

(For this discussion, I'm equating food quality with taste: does it have a bold, or otherwise satisfying flavor and/or texture? Not some bland same ol' same ol'. Someone else might rightly define food quality in terms of nutritional value, or production history as relates to food safety, or the humane treatment of animals. I won't quibble with anyone's definition of food quality, provided it harks back unto something inherent in the food itself, beyond mere economics. In other words, I challenge the notion that low cost, "value for the money," is a virtue when it comes to food, for reasons the text will make clear.)

Shouldn't energy balance be the priority regardless of how a food tastes?

To a point, of course. However, you will recall we said in Chapter 2 that all humans, all mammals in fact, feed in excess of need. It is not a character flaw to overeat, it is biology. Thus, consciously limiting energy intake for the purpose of permanently lowering one's BMI, while a start, will not in isolation often be a pathway to success. Rather, we must engage and manipulate ("fool" I phrased it earlier) that complex physiology that regulates energy balance and either prevents or maintains obesity, depending on where ones brain's "weight thermostat" happens to be set.

There are two parts to human brain activity involved in regulating energy balance and appetite. One part focuses on *energy homeostasis*, balancing the provision of energy substrates for metabolism. The other involves *hedonic*, or pleasure-seeking patterns of brain activity. To quote University of Pennsylvania School of Medicine researchers writing in the December 2008 *Endocrinology and Metabolism Clinics of North America*: "Appetite is also driven by factors beyond physiologic needs. Food provides powerful visual, smell, and taste signals which can override satiety and stimulate feeding."

I believe my strategy of fooling the brain into being satisfied with less, must out of necessity work on both components of brain appetite-regulating action: the energy-homeostasis part, and the hedonic part. That's where quality-not-quantity enters the equation. Better taste, aroma, appearance of food all satisfy our pleasure centers with less. Eat food of lower aesthetic quality, you'll end up eating more calories in the drive to satisfy the hedonic brain.

Looking at this quality food-and-beverage question in a more personal, less scientific way—I love to eat, and it would be enormously hypocritical of me to tell anyone, regardless of their BMI, not to love eating right alongside me. Accordingly, I never tell patients not to enjoy a treat, so long as the portion size, and frequency are reasonable with respect to their BMI, and their health status otherwise. In fact, the purpose of all this hand-ringing about weight is, largely, prevention of obesity-related diseases, with a resulting longer life span. But if a prerequisite for life prolongation is giving up the joys of life—*joie de vivre*—of eating a really good meal, sipping a good wine, or whatever floats your particular boat, some might ask, *why bother?* Quality of life is important; its importance compared to length of life (another *quality v. quantity* question) is a value judgment for each individual.

With respect to managing obesity, I can make good arguments for quality over quantity being a part of the path to success. Some of that involves manipulating hedonic brain activity, as discussed above. But there is more, beyond mere aesthetics, to food quality versus quantity that can be brought to bear on the whole question of the causes of the epidemic of obesity.

And anything related to cause, of course, might be related to solution. *Ergo, if we want to solve the obesity problem, we've first got to understand and solve the food-quality problem.*

A MUST READ

If you want to know the full story of what got us to this dismal place, read *Fat Land: How Americans Became the Fattest People in the World* (Houghton-Mifflin, 2003) by journalist Greg Crister.

I urge everyone to read this book.

The hardcover is 176 pages of entertaining text, excluding appendixes, referencing, and index. Crister shows how class, politics, culture, economics, and institutional lies (like the classic, "Don't be silly—everyone knows that it's the same as sugar," smack-down of a dissenter prior to the FDA's approval of high-fructose corn syrup) all have combined to make "Americans very fat, very fast." The cover art is worth the price of the book: a chubby baby, whose belly is a McDonald's hamburger, sitting on a map of the United States, pepperoni pizza slice in his fat little hands, surrounded by a variety of foods, having a scoop of ice cream with toppings shoved in its face by an adult female hand, presumably its mother.

I won't attempt to summarize *Fat Land*. Get it, read it. I will detail, however, two people whose stories Crister relates: (1) Earl Butz, powerful agriculture secretary under Presidents Nixon and Ford, and (2) David Wallerstein, one time movie-theater-chain executive, later a director of the McDonald's Corporation.

The "Rusty" Butz Effect

First, a personal reflection: Earl Butz was named Secretary of

Agriculture in 1971 and resigned in scandal, unrelated to anything we're discussing, in 1976. I was ten years old when he took office. How many, do you suppose, preadolescent and early teenage children, living as I was in a suburb of a medium-sized city—i.e., nowhere near a farm—can name the Secretary of Agriculture, much less recall him decades later?

Yet the name Earl Butz is one of my most vivid memories from that era's newscasts. He was constantly before cameras and in print. Granted, I was the son of a newspaper editor, more aware of current events than most my age, but I think the fact that I can remember the name Earl Butz to this day is remarkable, a testament to the man's power and influence.

On what?

Farm policy. Commodity import and export policy. Food prices. President Richard Nixon, facing a tough reelection, had brought Butz aboard to fix a crisis. Farmers, a Republican constituency, were failing financially and underproducing, all under the weight of poor weather, a devalued dollar, and government regulations, that for instance, required approval for large exports of commodities, such as grain. The results: food shortages, soaring prices of basic items, hamburger, cheese, sugar, margarine. Middle-class housewives went in revolt, literally. I well remember the great meat shortage of the early seventies. Butz to the rescue—he dumped the limits on export sales, brokered a huge grain sale to the starving Soviet Union (how well I remember *that* Cold War controversy), and encouraged surplus production of corn and soybeans, which due to the expanded overseas markets resulted in soaring farm income.

Butz then traveled to still-unstable Southeast Asia, post-Vietnam War, and machinated for low-tariff imports into the United States of Malaysian palm-tree oil, an incredibly unhealthy fat, more highly saturated than hog lard, which was sold to the American homemaker as nothing different than vegetable oil. It was cheap, abundant, tasted better than vegetable oil (because of its molecular similarity to lard!), and made anything last forever on supermarket shelves. Never mind the earliest American importers of the stuff called it axle grease. (Not an exaggeration—I recently learned palm oil was a major export from colonial West Africa, historians considering it the "lubricant of the industrial revolution.") Within months of Butz's Malaysia trip, McDonald's built an oil-processing plant there, for you see, frying in palm oil makes really tasty french fries. (This is the same government now assuming an increasingly greater role in running all our health care. I'm just sayin'...)

Palm oil was cheap and easy to use for the food and restaurant industries.

Fat problem solved.

What about the cost of cane sugar? Sugar prices made sweetening foods and beverages very expensive, made unnaturally high by an international pricing structure that was effectively a foreign-aid program for developing nations.

What about the cost of sugar...?

Butz's corn surpluses!

Along about 1971 food scientists in Japan invented high-fructose corn syrup (HFCS), which was cheap, six-times sweeter than cane sugar, and by the late 1970s enjoying all that Butz-inspired surplus corn as substrate for its mass production. Converting from cane sugar, Coke and Pepsi saved 20 percent in sweetener costs! And HFCS wasn't only usable in liquids. It prevented freezer burn in frozen foods, kept vending machine foods fresher tasting, and made packaged baked goods look as if just browned in the oven. (Chapter 15 puts a microscope on this major factor in epidemic of obesity and diabetes.)

Thanks largely to Earl "Rusty" Butz, by the early 1980s we faced no more shortages of meat, butter, sugar, or coffee. In their place we got a hyperabundance of cheap sugar and cheap fat, a boon to product development and sales for the convenience-food-and-beverage industry.

The significance of this sea change cannot be underestimated:

For the first time in human history, a general population had at its fingertips an almost limitless supply of inexpensive, tasty calories, which the economics of the industry could afford to package and sell profitably in ever larger portions.

The bomb was planted.

The fuse lit...

Supersizing

The other *Fat Land* figure I will speak of is McDonald's executive David Wallerstein, who innovated "supersizing," a marketing ploy wherein people get sold a lot more food, or drink, for very little more money. If the extra product is cheap enough, and sales brisk enough, the seller's profit margin balloons. It's the idea behind selling a large bucket of popcorn at the movies, for a very few dollars more than a tiny bag, which is in fact the setting in which Wallerstein first deployed this scheme. In doing so, he managed to overcame the public's aversion to the sin of gluttony, via enticing economics. Like a street-corner drug pusher, he hooked us on "value for the money."

The mantra of the unhealthy eater.

I implore you, I beg of you...

Ignore the marketing tactics of the food-and-restaurant industry.

Ignore deals.

I know, they sound like they're doing you a favor, but they're only trying to make more money. I want them to make money. I'm a capitalist from way back. I'm not saying they're doing anything wrong, just that we don't have to fall for it. They are not making you a deal to be nice; they are making you a deal to sell more product and beat out their competition. They are also not consciously, deliberately, trying to kill you. Or sabotage your BMI. Those are merely unintended consequences of their actions and the shortsightedness of the American consumer.

The Pause-and-Ponder Habit

I've said I will never begrudge anybody an enjoyable meal, or tasty treat, less so if the frequency and portions are reasonable. All I ask is that you pause a few seconds—that pausing, by the way, can become one of those habits I spoke about—pause and consider how whatever food or beverage you are considering fits in with the rest of your daily nutritional lifestyle plan. If you can make it fit, great, buy it and enjoy. If you decide to cheat, fine, cheat, just don't do it every day. But make even the cheating a *conscious decision.* Do not blunder along through life eating and drinking whatever happens to appear in the way of your mouth.

Think just for a moment about everything: the good, the bad, the right, the wrong. Make that a habit, a lifestyle. I'll bet you choose the good and the right at least a bit more often than the bad and the wrong—more so once you start to get some positive feedback from the bathroom scale, cholesterol levels, blood sugars, sense of wellbeing.

Anyway, in McDonald's or 7-Eleven or Red Lobster, wherever, make your decision, cheating or not, and stick with it. Base that decision, first, ideally, on nutritional and health considerations, with personal taste preferences a close second. Price, I recommend putting much lower down on the deciding-factor scale. Never base a food-and-drink-related decision only or primarily on price. If you have two alternatives, and one is healthier (lower calorie, higher quality) but you can't afford the healthier one, consider walking away. Do not ever eat or drink something you wouldn't choose for nutritional, health, or aesthetic reasons, just because of cost.

Don't misunderstand, I don't encourage buying something you can't afford just because it's healthier—that's a whole different personal-responsibility issue, living within your means, which is not our subject. There may not be a perfect solution in every situation. That's the nature of our existence and a reality we must navigate. All I ask is that you try to balance these issues best you can, and give these choices some real consideration, rather than allowing other stresses of life to steamroll over them. And try to tip your balance as much as possible toward health and quality, which should lead naturally to smaller portions, which may offset the higher cost anyway. If 500 calories of unhealthy Food A costs a dollar, and 250 calories of healthy Food B costs the same dollar, then buying Food B is the healthier choice, and you'll eat fewer calories, and you've paid no more than you would have choosing Food A, in spite of prioritizing factors other than cost.

Once your food-or-drink choice is made, however, hopefully on the right basis, do not let a marketing deal, change your mind.

Say no to the deal.

Stick to your guns.

TALES FROM THE WAR ON OBESITY

Let me illustrate with a true story, which occurred shortly after Tennessee Governor Bill Haslam, noting that over 1.5 million, one in three, Tennesseans were obese, made reducing this rate the target of his Health and Wellness Task Force. I was driving home late from my clinic and pulled into a gas station. After filling up my SUV I felt hungry and knew this business sold Krispy-Kreme donuts out of a case. I went inside, finding a few glazed treats remaining from that morning's delivery. I bagged one and went to the register, whereupon the cashier announced forcefully they were two for a dollar at that hour.

I replied, "I only want one."

Aghast, she said, "I'll have to charge you a dollar!"

I said that was fine.

Then added…

I'm serious, I did…

"That's why there's so much obesity—people, for example, eating two donuts instead of one."

"Save one for breakfast," she countered.

"Then I would eat a donut for breakfast instead of something healthier."

It was pretty clear she thought I was a lunatic.

I don't believe she had a clue where I was coming from—nor was this exchange driven by any arguably admirable mercantilistic fervor, a desire to increase her employer's profits. I was, in fact, insisting upon paying the same amount for *less* merchandise. I was a retailer's dream.

No, our exchange was symptomatic of that cashier, like a large swathe of the American public, *being brainwashed into believing getting more product for less money trumps everything!* She could not get her head around me positioning price at a lower priority level than eliminating even the possibility I might give in and eat two donuts instead of one.

I paid my dollar, and drove home eating one donut, cringing at the thought of government action—recalling the governor's initiative—restricting my choice to buy a donut (or two, or a dozen), or for that matter, a business's right to market products as they see fit. At this point it falls to the public to resist marketing pressures that foster overconsumption. If we can't, though, the government will do it for us. Is that what you want? I don't entirely oppose government action in this arena—perhaps financial incentives to promote healthier consumption, something like taxation of sweeteners and sugary beverages, and subsidies for water. I would just prefer to see us do it on our own. But whether by personal conviction, or by edict, healthy lifestyle choices must be prioritized over "value" and "cheap" if we are to claw ourselves out of this mess.

Other Examples

At Cracker Barrel, I ordered pancakes, bacon, coffee. Period. My server—knowing not what she did—pointed out some menu item that added eggs to what I had ordered, which was cheaper than what my order would come to. "No thanks," I said politely, but firmly, omitting the obesity-epidemic lecture this time.

She smiled and went off.

Saying "no" to these situations is an ingrained habit for me.

It needs to become so for you, too.

And—I kid you not—I had an almost repeat of the donut incident on another late-night trip home, another gas station, this one selling two-for-one hot dogs! This exchange was with another customer, a friendly guy looking like Ben Vereen. He absolutely could not believe I wouldn't get a second hot dog. Then, I have to admit, he said something that made me cave: "Get two and give it to the dog." Well, as it happens, on these late nights I habitually give Emma, the large blonde dog living in a plastic igloo on our patio, a snack when I get home. My price of admittance, I guess. That night Emma snarfed down a hot dog. Hopefully the Humane Society isn't putting me on a list, but in my defense, I only fell for the marketing ploy when it otherwise fit with an established/intentional lifestyle habit—in this case, giving the dog a snack. And before you say it, I promise no homeless person was in the immediate vicinity to receive the surplus hot dog.

Speaking of homeless people, I'll tell one more story. Last one, I promise, and I'm almost ashamed to admit this one too involves Krispy-Kreme donuts. My wife and I had doctor's appointments in downtown Nashville and arrived early. We walked a number of blocks (a healthy lifestyle habit!) to the Krispy-Kreme joint across from Baptist Hospital. We each got coffee and I (my wife is a better person than me naturally) ordered one glazed donut. We turned down samples offered us across the counter. Outside, walking back to where we needed to be, I looked in my bag and there were two donuts inside. I ate one and woke up a homeless man sleeping on the front steps of a church and gave him the bag with the other one in it. "That's for you," I told him, and walked away. My mother always said, "There's more than one way to skin a cat." There too is more than one way to avoid overeating.

In telling these tales I don't claim to be any paragon of nutritional virtue. I was not eating "healthy" on those occasions, although with moderation, anybody can get away with almost anything from time to time. My point is, there are simple steps we can take to mitigate the impact of marketing on our efforts to eat healthy. The American food and restaurant industries excel at adding unnecessary calories to our meals. When was the last time you ate at a sit-down restaurant and didn't get a basket of bread? And don't most restaurant breakfasts automatically include toast or muffins? But you can get into the habit of proactively asking for no bread.

And we should all be in the habit of saying "no" to specials.

But Dr. Rone, do you pay full price for marked-down items in, say, a clothing store?

Of course not.

Special pricing, however, in food-and-beverage retailing is a plague best avoided. In a clothing store, if I buy one shirt and get a second free, what's the harm? That's different from two-for-one pricing for a food item, in which *harm is done*. My calorie intake increases, which, in 21st century America, equals harm until proven otherwise.

Now, if the shirt deal is, say, buy one, get half off another, that's different. If you would have bought the second shirt anyway, great. If the deal allows you to get an extra shirt you really do need but couldn't have afforded, that's great too. But if you're only buying it because of the deal, I *would* think twice. You're lightening your wallet or checking account, or increasing your credit-card balance, and I *would* argue you shouldn't do that for pricing reasons alone. Obviously that advice is outside the scope of this book; I mention it only to illustrate another parallel between weight management and personal-financial management.

For sure though, when it comes to calorie intake, beware of marketing that aims to increase profit by putting more food in your stomach. It is ubiquitous. It is everywhere, we ignore it, we take it for granted, like background noise.

Don't.

Stop. Think. Say no. Be your own calorie-purchase boss.

Resistance is not futile.

THE IMPOVERISHED?

Many people struggle to make ends meet, are perhaps out of work, feeding a large family. It might seem I am unsympathetic, or oblivious, especially as I press ahead here, encouraging a willingness to pay more for better quality. That may come across as a very nice, yet elitist idea.

I will point out, however, that obesity, and most lifestyle diseases, like diabetes, hit the lower socioeconomic groups in America worse than the higher ones. Not just America—2010 data analyzed by researchers at the Harvard School of Public Health linked 180,000 deaths per year worldwide to sugar-sweetened beverages, and 78 percent of those deaths were in low- and middle-income countries. So while my advice might be harder for a low-income family to follow, it is no less relevant to that family, and may be more so. I would ask the mom in Walmart contemplating a "super-value pack" of snacks for her kids' lunch boxes to consider how much is really being saved, compared to buying a smaller pack of something healthier, or lower calorie, or made from better ingredients, but costing a little more per ounce.

If the more expensive purchase means each child gets a smaller portion, that might be for the best—remember "portion distortion." And remember, the epidemic of obesity has in no way spared our children.

(I've always thought it ironic that in times past, the very poor literally starved—were skin-and-bones malnourished—while in our modern society of abundance, the very poor are more likely to be obese that the rest of us! Case in point, a newspaper article and accompanying photo a few days before Thanksgiving, about a local church giving away holiday turkeys to needy families. The write-up quoted a mother saying, "How hard is it not to have enough to feed your family? It's hard." The photo showed her appreciatively receiving her food box, and I don't believe 300 pounds to be an overestimate of her weight. I don't suggest she wasn't deserving, nor that she was doing anything underhanded, or failing to care for her children. But the scenario spoke volumes to me about our food industry and retailing—the underappreciated effect of focusing on cost over quality—and the impact of nebulous factors like education and lifestyle and stress on the epidemic of obesity.)

This is a good place to acknowledge that *nothing in this book is meant to address or pontificate about abject poverty.* The person who truly does not know where his or her next meal is coming from, who is underweight, skin and bones as a result, is pointedly not the subject of this book, nor target for my advice. This book is about treating obesity and struggling to avoid obesity. Period. Its focus is of course medical, not socioeconomic, but to the extent that socioeconomic factors influence this medical problem strongly, I am obligated to try to address those points as best I can.

13

BETTER FOOD QUALITY: HOW & WHY?

Most of us would agree, for any product category, choosing the lower-cost alternative, probably also means buying lower quality. No doubt there are exceptions, but generally speaking that is an economic reality, perhaps *necessity*. You get what you pay for. I would argue, though, that one product category where it is almost always better to spend whatever it takes to get the highest quality you can possibly afford is the food-product category.

We are what we eat.

Do you really want to go out of your way to buy the cheapest food and drink for yourself and your family—the stuff that fuels our days, makes our brains think, hydrates our cells, provides the protein to grow and maintain our muscles, the fats that sheath our nerve fibers. Do you really want to load your body and your family's bodies with chemicals used by the food industry to promote mass production, long-distance shipping, extended shelf life? The hormones and antibiotics that grow food animals like chickens and cattle at unnaturally rapid rates, protect them from disease in unnaturally (and cruelly) dense living conditions? The insecticides and herbicides and genetic modifications that grow our wheat and other plant-food products more rapidly, with higher yields?

Just asking?

ISN'T FOOD INSPECTED AND TESTED?

I'm not trying to sound like a crazed survivalist here—there's much hype on both sides of the food-safety issue—but I think it common sense to avoid consuming to the extent possible extra chemicals that

God and/or Mother Nature didn't intend for us. The US Food and Drug Administration (FDA) can tell us a food additive is safe, approving it for human consumption but, to be blunt, I will never fully believe them.

Case in point:

The 1976 Toxic Substances Control Act is widely considered to be a joke, according to Tom Ashbrook, on National Public Radio's *On Point* broadcast of 5/30/13. Of roughly 85,000 chemicals registered for use in the United States, only two hundred have been tested by the Environmental Protection Agency (EPA), and only five have been banned—since 1976!

Now, to be clear, this data relates to the work of the EPA, tasked with protecting us from environmental exposures, such as cancer-causing dioxin, not deliberately ingested exposures in the form of food and beverages. That is the purview of the FDA and the USDA. I'm simply using the data presented on NPR to illustrate a general point:

Anybody depending 100 percent on, trusting 100 percent, a government bureaucracy to watch over their wellbeing, is a fool. Let me repeat, and I am very serious, a fool. Again, not trying to sound like an anti-government wacko, but if you think the FDA and the USDA and the EPA have required and scrutinized (or ever could) sufficient research on every chemical the American food supply is exposed to, in every possible combination, to confirm that human consumption over a lifetime is safe, then I've got about five bridges to sell you. I didn't say *absolutely safe*. Nothing is 100 percent. I'm saying it is impossible to prove even reasonable safety, under real-world conditions, over decades of exposure, without the sort of long-term, large-sample research no commercial concern is ever going to fund or wait for when trying to bring a product to market. And that's fine; there are many products I wouldn't want to wait that long for. I'm just saying our food-safety watchdogs can only do so much.

I trust them to make sure nothing meant for my consumption, on the shelf at my local Publix, is immediately or subacutely poisonous. Beyond that, without being paranoid, we have to use common sense, think, educate ourselves, make discriminating choices. Take personal

---

* If the reference is lost on you, see the 1973 film *Soylent Green*, the title referring to a government-distributed food product (the ingredients of which are a little murky, but they taste really good) fed to an overpopulated United States. Based on the late Harry Harrison's 1966 novel *Make Room! Make Room!*.

responsibility. We are intelligent human beings, not cattle, nor dogs, eating whatever is stuck in front of us.

Remember...

"Soylent Green is people."*

The Ultimate Test

So, how *do* we make reasonably sure what we're eating and drinking is safe if consumed regularly for years? The only experiment that can do justice to that question is the "real-life" experiment: *What has proven reasonably safe, or not unduly harmful, over years, decades, generations, of real-world experience?*

The answer to that question is, for once, easy—most anything and everything people have actually been eating and drinking for years, decades, generations. In fact, if you couple ancient, or pre-modern food and beverage choices, with a few basic modern techniques to prevent spoilage and contamination, like refrigeration, cooking with adequate heat, safe drinking water, then you've really got something.

There is an ilk of diet book based on ancient food choices—*The Maker's Diet* and *The Paleolithic Diet*, being examples—based on the notion I am presenting. Michael Pollan, a journalist and "liberal foodie intellectual," wrote in *New York Times Magazine* in 2007:

> Don't eat anything your great-great-grandmother wouldn't recognize as food. (Sorry, but at this point Moms are as confused as the rest of us, which is why we have to go back a couple of generations, to a time before the advent of modern food products.)

This boils down to, for lack of a better term, eat *naturally*, eat so-called *whole foods*. Choosing certified-organic products is one way to avoid certain additives and bastardizations (think Twinkie) of the modern food industry, but don't trust wholeheartedly that one label—that too is abdicating personal responsibility—nor do you need to limit yourself to foods labeled *organic*. Read labels. Use common sense. Employ Pollan's Great-Great-Grandmother Rule. Look for statements like: "no hormones," "no antibiotics," "grass-fed," rather than "corn-fed." (Corn isn't wholly evil, but it is the substrate of much that is bad in the modern food industry.) Scrutinize fine-print ingredients lists on food labels. The longer the list, the less natural, more processed, less healthy, a product is likely to be. A long list of things sounding pretty simple and natural in and of themselves might be okay, but short lists are reassuring. And the more things you can't pronounce, much less explain, the more wary you should be.

One ingredient I scan for—get in that *habit*, too, scan the labeling of everything you buy—is high-fructose corn syrup (HFCS). If something is supposed to have sugar in it, I want to see "sugar" on the label, which I take to mean cane sugar, or sucrose. If it's got HFCS instead, I usually put it back. We'll have the come-to-Jesus lecture on HFCS chapter after next. Suffice to say for now, it's a red flag for something that ain't even trying to appear natural.

Is "Natural" Always Better?

When it comes to food and drink, *natural* is not a bad way to describe the stuff that is generally best to select. A truly natural food, provided it isn't covered in dirt and botulism toxin, is probably safer and healthier than a purely synthetic or highly processed food. As a concept then, *natural*—meaning less processed, less adulterated, not created from scratch in a factory, sold and consumed in largely the same form it was harvested or slaughtered in, perhaps in relatively close geographic proximity to the place it was harvested or slaughtered—is a useful path to good nutrition and health.

The word *natural* though gets batted around an awful lot in the labeling and marketing of all sorts of food and non-food products, and of it, you must be wary. There is a pervasive, and wrong assumption that anything "natural" must by definition be safe—or at least safer, and better than something non-natural.

Natural, let's be clear, is not, never has been, a synonym for *safe*.

Curare is extracted from South American plants; it's as natural as anything, and it's deadly poison.

I've had many discussions with patients about thyroid-hormone replacement products, a focus of my practice. Many are convinced natural thyroid supplements, like Armour Thyroid, extracted from actual pig thyroid glands, is better, safer, more effective than synthetic, factory-produced alternatives, like Synthroid. That simply isn't true for most people. Besides, the most abundant active ingredient in Armour Thyroid is the same molecule as the active ingredient in Synthroid.

I recently diagnosed a patient as a laxative abuser. She countered that what she was doing was okay because she was very careful to only buy a "natural laxative." A moment's online research told me the product she was using was, indeed, manufactured from a natural source of the active ingredient in Senokot—one of the harshest laxatives you can buy. It made absolutely no difference that her laxative was natural; it had the same effect on her body that a similar synthetic product would, yet there was no convincing my patient of that. I insisted she stop and she did. She stopped coming to see me, that is.

Do. Not. Listen. To. Hype.

Think for yourself. If a food product is labeled *natural*, don't buy it solely for that reason. Scrutinize the label as much as you would for anything, understand what you're getting, and evaluate how that fits into your nutritional plans and goals.

DEPLOYING QUALITY VS. QUANTITY IN YOUR STRUGGLE

With respect to weight management, if you spend more on higher-quality, less-processed, less-mass-produced foods, I believe you will eat less, and have a better BMI and lower blood sugar as a result.

Why?

First—not everything has to be complicated—if you spend more per item or per quantity, then you probably aren't going to buy as much, and what you don't buy, you can't eat.

The opposite also holds. Buy cheaper, value foods, you'll buy more, making more calories readily available to be dished out to your family and eaten. Consider: $10 worth of chicken, versus $10 worth of potato chips.

Now, you could argue that just because a certain quantity is purchased doesn't mean it has be prepared all at once, or served all at once, or you have to eat it all at once. You can stop yourself and have leftovers, an excellent strategy when all else fails. But let's face it, if it is on your plate there's a darn good chance you'll eat it, and if it's on the stove, it's only a little less likely you'll get up and serve yourself seconds.

If you are serious about cutting calories, far better there be no excess calories in the house, on the stove, for sure not on the plate. Convenience, efficiency, stocking the cupboard, fixing extra for later: are all the enemy of nutritional management. If you don't want to eat it, don't have it in reach.

For it is fundamentally against human nature—human survival instinct—not to eat what's available. I also think there is something else going on, beyond the simple fact it's harder to overbuy expensive items.

Our bodies need satisfaction.

They crave it.

I introduced this concept last chapter under the term *hedonic brain activity*. The more high quality the food is, the tastier it is, the more carefully (even lovingly) prepared it is, the more your great-great-grandmother would recognize it as food, rather than an agglutination of chemicals, the more it will satisfy—that is, trigger those stop-eating signals, and suppress those hedonic eat-more signals.

Eat lower quality foods, though, and you'll have to eat more calories before needed satisfaction levels are achieved. The quintessence of our value-for-the-money food culture is the scene where a typical American couple is dining in some haute cuisine restaurant and the waiter with great aplomb serves a big plate with a tiny amount of beautifully arranged food in the middle, and the couple looks with dismay at each other. Next scene, of course, they're fleeing into McDonald's or Shoney's or Pizza Hut and stuff themselves silly.

That mentality, make no mistake…

Explains the epidemic of obesity.

14

UNREAL SWEETENERS, PART I

This chapter and the next continue the quality-not-quantity theme, but focus on the specific issue of how (and *how much!*) we sweeten our foods and beverages. There are two broad topics here, and it wouldn't be inappropriate to lump both under the rubric *artificial sweeteners*. The first involves what are often called *artificial*, but should more properly be called *non-caloric sweeteners*.

The second deals with *high-fructose corn syrup*: most definitely artificial, and caloric.

BLUE AND PINK STUFF

Non-caloric sweeteners in widespread use in the United States include saccharin (Sweet'N Low, which comes in those little pink single-serving packets), aspartame (NutraSweet and Equal, the latter coming in those little blue packets), sucralose (Splenda), and stevia (Truvia and others). Stevia is the only one of theses not synthetically produced, being extracted from a South American herb. And while they are used in other ways—sucralose can sweeten baked goods, for example—by far the largest use of these chemicals is in the sweetening of "diet sodas," about which I have a number of concerns.

Most basic of these concerns is my own observation that, in spite of what would appear to be massive use of diet-soda products—judging from how much space they take up on grocery shelves—there has been no abatement of the obesity and diabetes epidemics. In fact, my own diabetes control and weight have *improved* since I stopped drinking diet soda—without even completely purging real sodas from my diet!

Granted, I've made other changes, but I'm not the only one observing this confusing phenomenon, which I will call the *diet-soda paradox.*

I have already quoted Dr. Jon Ebbert of the Mayo Clinic (see Chapter 10) as arguing that, in so many words, low- or no-calorie sweeteners help perpetuate an appetite for sweetness that carries forward, leading to greater future calorie, and in particular sugar-calorie consumption.

A large study completed in 2007 showed that drinking one or more diet sodas per day *increased* the risk of developing diabetes by 67 percent. Studies link diet soda to kidney disease and metabolic syndrome, and those looking at the effectiveness of these products in weight management are conflicting. Two observational studies, published in 2008 and 2012, show consumption of artificially sweetened beverages was followed by weight gain. Other studies have shown weight loss, or no change. Some (like Dr. Ebbert) believe diet soda directly stimulates appetite, increasing cravings for carbohydrates, leading to T2DM, metabolic syndrome, and weight gain. Others blame human behavior, rather than physiology—if we are "saving" calories by drinking diet soda then we give ourselves permission to eat other high-calorie foods.

My belief is two fold:

One, anybody who drinks a lot of soda, diet or not, has unhealthy habits, which in and of themselves lead to diabetes, metabolic syndrome, and obesity. And two, I believe the ingestion of sweet liquids not associated with actual calorie intake confuses the brain's appetite and satiety centers, such that natural, instinctual limits on food consumption are hobbled. This is an extension of my *our-bodies-need-satisfaction theory.* At a minimum, the *diet-soda paradox* (the lack of obvious, wide-spread improvements in obesity and diabetes with sugar-free-soda use) is consistent with the realization that appetite and energy balance in humans is far more complex than we have naïvely believed.

For example, there are sweet-taste receptors in the wall of the small intestine—who'da thought?—identical to those on the tongue. These receptors are linked to the release of "fullness" signals, like GLP-1. A 2012 paper in *Diabetes Care*, tantalizingly, documented differences in how various liquids interacted with these intestinal taste buds, and how those interactions differed in type 2 diabetics compared to normal individuals. Specifically, in diabetics, diet soda failed to trigger those signals—meaning that, in diabetes at least, diet soda fails to satisfy the appetite, potentially promoting further consumption, further weight gain, and worsening diabetes control, compared to what might've resulted, ironically, from drinking a true sugary beverage.

The diet-soda paradox indicates that *regulating appetite and satiety signals might be more important to weight-management than simple calorie reduction.* Diet sodas help the later, but not universally the former. Which, in so many words, is an overarching theme of this book: that on the one hand weight loss is as simple as cutting energy intake to less than expenditure, yet, in order to make that arithmetic work, other tricks need to be played to "fool" our appetites, to not only make it easier—but perhaps to make it even possible. And diet soda doesn't play the trick we need it to, which might be more impactful in a negative way than its lack of calories is in a positive one.

There is even speculation that these intestinal sweet-taste receptors regulate the speed and amount of absorption of real glucose—thus, diet soda consumed with a meal might trigger more rapid and robust absorption of glucose contained in the meal, raising blood sugars, and increasing insulin spikes, promoting obesity and poor diabetes control.

The American Diabetes and American Heart Associations opined jointly in August 2012 with a scientific statement titled "Nonnutritive Sweeteners: Current Use and Health Perspectives." They concluded: "At this time, there are insufficient data to determine conclusively whether the use of [nonnutritive sweeteners]…benefits appetite, energy balance, body weight, or cardiometabolic risk factors."

A Thyroid-Diet Soda Connection?

There was an intriguing case report at the 2013 American Association of Clinical Endocrinologists meeting opening up a whole new concern about diet sodas. It described a heavy consumer of artificial sweeteners who was diagnosed and treated for Hashimoto's thyroiditis, an immune-system disorder commonly causing hypothyroidism. Her thyroid disease was unusual because she had no family history and no other evidence of immune disease. When she stopped all sugar substitutes, however, her thyroid levels—which had started out low, then become normal on treatment—all of a sudden became high. When her thyroid medication was stopped her levels returned to normal, and stayed normal. She currently has no evidence of Hashimoto's thyroiditis.

This is one report, one person, and may not hold true for the broader swath of the American public. However, if non-caloric sweeteners do trigger low thyroid levels in some people, they put users at risk of the whole gamut of metabolic derangements, including weight gain and fatigue, including lipid disorders, even a promotion of heart disease that is associated with hypothyroidism.

A final concern I have about non-calorie sweeteners, besides their unclear efficacy achieving the goals that are the only conceivable rationale for their use, is that they are yet another class of largely synthetic chemicals being poured into our food supply by the bucketsful. The most controversial of these substances is *aspartame*, whose safety has long been debated. I won't attempt to pass judgment, except to say that too much of most things isn't good. A small amount of aspartame is probably fine; large amounts I have concerns about. And remember, it is best to be skeptical about the safety of any additives, including non-caloric sweeteners, which have not long (generations long) been part of the human food chain.

15

UNREAL SWEETENERS, PART II:
FRANKEN-SUGAR?

High-fructose corn syrup: industry loves it. It's inexpensive, easy to transport, keeps foods moist. It's six times sweeter than cane sugar, meaning smaller quantities are needed to get the same taste. From a practical standpoint, let's face it, HFCS is here to stay. Is it really, then, gram for gram, the horrible awful ogre of food additives all the negative publicity and my own foregoing comments would imply?

Well...

Yes and *No*.

It is handled differently, in medically problematic ways, than other sugars. In other respects, though, it isn't all that different from other sugars. It contains four calories per gram like all sugars, for example, and therefore many concerns we have about it aren't so much unique to HFCS, but generally applicable to all sugar and carbohydrate intake.

And there is a lot of concern about that.

Sugar consumption has risen 40 fold since the Declaration of Independence was signed. According to Harvard nutritionist Mary Franz, Americans ingest 130 pounds of sugar per year, an average of 38 teaspoons per day (the American Heart Association advising no more than six to nine per day). And more than a third of that added sugar is in the form of soft drinks, or other sweetened beverages, mostly sweetened with HFCS. And some so-called fruit juices, remember, contain HFCS. It's also in pancake syrups, popsicles, yogurts, ketchup, BBQ sauces, pasta sauces, soups, breakfast cereals, the list goes on.

So, if we are ingesting too much sugar, and the majority of ingested sugar is HFCS, then HFCS is the biggest contributor to the excess-sugar problem. But: is HFCS a problem separate from the sugar problem in general? It does have one unique property causing it to single-handedly expand the sugar problem:

Its cheapness.

Industry gets more value for its money with HFCS than cane sugar.

There's that vile word again:

Value.

HFCS, no question, is part and parcel of our "quality versus quantity" issue. HFCS availability has promoted the packaging and marketing of sweetened products in irresponsibly large quantities, fostering in turn the purchasing and consuming of these products in irresponsibly large quantities. If, however, we reined in all this irresponsibility, where might that leave our critical assessment of HFCS?

FRUCTOSE 101

Fructose is not Frankenstein food. It is a naturally occurring *monosaccharide*, or simple sugar. It is a major sugar in many fruits, and makes up half of the mass of a molecule of cane sugar, aka *sucrose*, which is a *disaccharide*, two monosaccharides linked by a molecular bond. The simple sugars joining to form sucrose are one six-carbon fructose and one six-carbon glucose. Fructose is the most abundant sugar in honey, and makes up about half the sugar by weight in molasses. Maple syrup is almost all sucrose, meaning it's half fructose. Regular old corn syrup is all glucose, and starchy foods—potatoes, beans and lentils, wheat, rice, oats—all break down to release pure glucose.

So, from a broad perspective, a diet heavy on potatoes, legumes, and grains is supplying glucose as the major carbohydrate, while one heavy on fruits and added sweets, like table sugar, syrups, molasses, and honey are getting roughly a 50:50 mix of fructose and glucose.

Obviously, then, a balanced diet, even a relatively natural and healthy one, even before the advent of HFCS, contained fructose in some significant ratio relative to glucose.

A History of Dietary Fructose: the Good, Bad, and Ugly

Let's invent a hypothetical 1950s diet wherein half the carbohydrates are from the potatoes/legumes/grains category and half are from the fruits/sweets category. That would yield a simple sugar intake of about 75 percent glucose and 25 percent fructose. Now, the brain and muscles are the principal fuel consumers of the body. The brain, in an average man, accounts for 25 percent of total calories burned. And except under unusual circumstances, the brain only uses glucose. Muscle uses a mix of glucose, fats, and ketones.

Notice: *Was fructose mentioned?*

Fructose cannot be directly used as a fuel by the body.

More on that later.

Anyway, this hypothetical 1950s carb intake, remember, was 75 percent glucose (which can be directly burned) and 25% fructose (which can't).

Jump to today…

My guess is we're still consuming a lot of glucose in the form of grains, maybe potatoes, but less in the form of vegetables. There is more sweet stuff these days, much of it sugary foods and beverages (soft drink consumption has increased five fold since 1950), and those carbs are at least 50:50 fructose-to-glucose, and remember HFCS is an additive in many foods you wouldn't expect, cheaper mayonnaise brands, for instance, and white bread. Now, I'm guessing, but say the modern diet relative to the 1950s would shift the mostly-glucose (starch) portion to about 30 percent and the fruits/sweet 50:50 fructose:glucose portion to 70 percent. Using those assumptions, the arithmetic gives us a modern carbohydrate intake of around 65 percent glucose and 35 percent fructose (compared to 75 and 25, respectively, in the fifties). That may not seem like much of a shift, except when you consider the portion of carb calories that can't be directly used as fuel (i.e., fructose) has increased by 40 percent!

Now, before even looking at the accumulating research, I'm going to spitball what that might mean for the modern average American compared to the 1950s average American. The modern American having 40 percent more carb calories not directly utilizable by the body:

- Fatigue/weakness/poor concentration at work or school?

- Increased appetite, driving greater calorie consumption, trying to make up the loss?

- "Desperation" metabolism of fructose to dig out those four calories per gram? (I didn't say fructose was calorie free, I said it couldn't be *directly* burned.)

- In the process of that "desperation" metabolism, might there be "metabolic exhaust," like a car burning oil? (Indeed, yes, and I'll give you a hint—it's fat!)

Enter High-Fructose Corn Syrup

Okay, as we put the role of fructose in our diets into historical perspective, let's pause now to explain what exactly is HFCS.

The compound adjective "high-fructose" is, truthfully, misleading. It is only there to distinguish HFCS from regular corn syrup, which is all glucose. In fact, the version of HFCS used in beverages in the United States, *HFCS 55*, is 52 percent fructose and 42 percent glucose. Another form, *HFCS 42*—42 percent fructose, 52 percent glucose—is used in various prepared foods. Thus, HFCS really isn't, gram for gram, much worse than cane sugar, which is half and half, fructose and glucose. The reality of the above cited proportions in the composition of HFCS has been challenged, however. A letter in the 1/17/13 issue of *The New England Journal of Medicine* argued the mix of glucose and fructose in HFCS was "varying and unregulated," citing a 2011 paper in which Ventura et al. reported popular sugar-sweetened beverages had double the fructose compared to glucose. It also may be that free fructose and free glucose dissolved suspension, as comprises HFCS, may be more unhealthy and obesity promoting than glucose and fructose bound molecularly in the form of sucrose, consumed as a disaccharide, requiring additional digestion.

I believe those to be valid concerns. And there are others about the chemistry of HFCS, about how its fructose component is handled by the body, which we will discuss shortly. I think the *economics* of HFCS, however, is at least as big a problem, perhaps bigger, than its *chemistry*. As I said in this chapter's introduction, HFCS is cheap, and versatile. It has been widely adapted by the food-and-beverage industry, fueling expanded product lines, and changing consumer habits, such that a greater percentage of our calories today are carbohydrates, than once was the case, and a greater percentage of our carbohydrates are fructose.

It is unfortunate, and no more than a coincidence, that the rise of HFCS overlapped with a completely different driver of changing nutritional habits, something completely distinct from food-industry economics:

Public health education, the medical profession and federal officials promoting for decades an overly simplified, endlessly pervasive, drumming message that, essentially, fats were bad, and carbohydrates were good.

That campaign culminated in what was, in my opinion, *one of the greatest public-health blunders, perhaps catastrophes, in the history of the United States Government*:

The 1992 Food Guide Pyramid.

For a full discussion of the weaknesses of and ideas for revision of the "food pyramid," which was subsequently modified for the better, I recommend *Eat, Drink, and Be Healthy* by Dr. Walter Willett, of the Harvard School of Public Health. For our purposes, let me just remind you, the original food pyramid placed as its base— symbolizing the foundation of a healthy diet, where most calories should come from—breads, cereals, rice, pasta (all carbs).

Fruits and vegetables (also carb heavy) made up the next higher, smaller tier.

The much smaller top half of the pyramid consisted of dairy foods, meats, beans, eggs, nuts, fats, oils, and sweets, in roughly that descending order of advised consumption.

This highly publicized, oft-published icon of nutritional education further brainwashed the public that all fats were bad and most carbs were good. By this point of course, we were well into the HFCS era, which saw, according to my ciphering above, a possibly 40 percent increase in the relative amount of fructose compared to glucose in the carbohydrate portion of the American diet. That, coupled with the food pyramid promoting a bloating of the carbohydrate portion of the average diet, plus the message going back to the 1950s from doctors and the government to limit meat and fat (indirectly screaming: Eat carbs!), produced in the 1990s a perfect storm of obesity-generating nutrition:

Carb laden.

Fructose heavy.

It Gets Worse

I assume the original food pyramid's creators honestly thought they were bringing to bear, on an important public-health concern, the best nutritional science and thought leadership available. I do think it folly to seek one set of recommendations for all 300 million genetically diverse Americans, but be that as it may, I'll grant them that benefit of the doubt.

I believe however that *we*—I finished my endocrine training in 1992, the year the food pyramid was born, so I share responsibility, to the extent that I too promoted its message to my patients in the beginning—we overlooked, however inadvertently, two critical factors:

- The metabolic impact of fructose, and...
- The impact of insulin resistance

An understanding of insulin resistance, a major contributor to the pathophysiology of diabetes, was just beginning to permeate mainstream medicine at that time, but certainly not Washington politics, a major shaper (pun intended) of the food pyramid—the seminal paper on insulin resistance, having been delivered by Dr. Ralph DeFronzo, then of Yale, now of the University of Texas-San Antonio, in 1987 to the American Diabetes Association, in his Banting Award lecture.

More to come on insulin resistance. For now, suffice it to say, it renders a person intolerant to carbohydrates, the excess intake of which, in these people in particular, leads to obesity, diabetes, hypertension, hyperlipidemia, heart disease, stroke.

And death.

Not a good thing at a time when the food industry, and healthcare, and the federal government were all ganging up, marching to the drumbeat:

High-carb, low-fat, rah, rah, rah!

FRUCTOSE BIOCHEMISTRY AND PHYSIOLOGY

The human handling of fructose, how it differs from glucose, is a complex subject—more so than even I thought going into this. For example, intestinal-lining cells convert some absorbed fructose into glucose. I have found conflicting information on how much fructose is converted in this manner, but it might be quite low in humans compared to other animals. Certainly this would not likely be a robust, efficient process for dealing with the large amounts of ingested fructose existing today.

Glucose and Fructose Assimilation

The rate of passage of fructose from gut to bloodstream is about half that of glucose. Glucose is absorbed by a complex series of events, consisting of energy-driven *active transport*, and *facilitated diffusion*— glucose piggybacked onto a protein linked to the vigorous movement of sodium into blood capillaries. Fructose transport is not linked to sodium, nor any energy-burning process. The slower absorption of fructose has been used to argue that it might be the preferred sugar for patients with diabetes, some of whose problems relate to after-meal spikes in blood sugar. Also, fructose utilization, such as it is, is independent of insulin, potentially getting around the insulin deficiency/resistance issues diabetics deal with.

Neither argument has practical validity. The brain cannot use fructose. It uses glucose almost exclusively and does not require insulin. Muscles can't use fructose either, but can readily use fatty acids, which we will see, fructose can be turned into. The overuse of fatty acids as a fuel source may cause ketoacidosis, a life-threatening diabetes complication. So, fructose, by itself, is not a better alternative to glucose in anybody, including a diabetic. In fact, laboratory animals whose liver and intestines have been removed, die from hypoglycemia if only fructose is infused intravenously.

Cellular Metabolism

Once in the bloodstream both glucose and fructose travel to the liver. Glucose passes right through, reaching the heart, which pumps it to the rest of the body, but predominantly to brain and muscle cells. Once inside a cell, glucose undergoes *glycolysis*, a sequence of chemical reactions, whereby the six-carbon glucose molecule is metabolized, releasing some energy, to form the two-carbon molecule *acetyl-CoA*.

Glycolysis serves two functions: (1) energy release in the form of a chemical called *ATP*, and (2) the provision of carbon skeletons, for the synthesis of everything the body needs, including amino acids for protein building, and nucleic acids for chromosome building.

Not all consumed glucose is burned immediately by glycolysis. Glycolysis is, in fact, tightly regulated, and the enzyme *phosphofructokinase* (PFK) is its control switch. An enzyme is a protein that facilitates a biochemical reaction, in this case, one of the ten steps that make up the process of glycolysis. Anything that slows the PFK reaction will result in fewer glucose molecules being burned by glycolysis, whereas a lack of any such PFK inhibitor will cause more glucose to be burned. PFK is inhibited by: (1) ATP, the body's main energy currency—the presence of which says the body has plenty of energy and doesn't need more—and (2) *citrate*, a signal that the body has enough of those biosynthetic building blocks, what we called carbon skeletons above. If PFK is blocked by adequate energy and adequate building blocks, glucose cannot be converted to acetyl CoA and it gets stored instead as glycogen—a readily accessible, nonfatty, glucose store found in the liver and muscles.

Fructose, on the other hand, is stopped dead in the liver.

It is converted there to fructose-1-phosphate—which, in turn, enters normal glycolysis by three different routes, all of which bypass PFK, the major control point.

Thus, fructose unregulatedly—think, undisciplinedly—is metabolized in the liver to acetyl-CoA. No opportunity for ATP or citrate to have their say, to determine whether carbohydrate is to be burned, or else stored responsibly as glycogen. All fructose is turned blithely into acetyl-CoA.

So? What's wrong with acetyl-CoA?

Have you ever even heard of it?

Bet not.

Yet...

Acetyl-CoA is the central substance in all human metabolism.

It's like, "Absolute power corrupts absolutely." You want to handle it responsibly, like metabolic dynamite, and taking in excess fructose and unregulatedly making excess acetyl-CoA is like having a wild orangutan throwing your dynamite all over the place.

What's Special About Acetyl-CoA?

Acetyl-CoA (ACoA) lies at the crossroads of all the major metabolic pathways. The energy-releasing breakdown of nearly all carbohydrate and fat molecules form ACoA. Many amino acids form ACoA as well when proteins are degraded. So, to one degree or another, all foodstuffs are digested to ACoA, and once formed, ACoA has several possible fates.

One is to enter the *Krebs cycle* to be oxidized to carbon dioxide (CO_2), which travels to the lungs to be exhaled. The Krebs cycle releases electrons which throw off more ATP energy units during *oxidative phosphorylation*, the process that ultimately transfers those electrons to oxygen inhaled by the lungs. Oxygen (O_2) combines with hydrogen to form water (H_2O). Thus, out of all this we get the basic equation of carbohydrate metabolism: *Glucose* + O_2 = CO_2 + H_2O. One molecule of glucose releasing 36 ATP molecules in the process. This is the main energy-generating pathway taken by ACoA.

Another possible ACoA fate is ketone-body production. These are useful fuels during emergencies, like starvation or heavy physical exertion, but can become deadly poisons in some diabetics. ACoA, also via the Kreb's cycle, goes into the synthesis of amino acids for protein and nucleic-acid (DNA and RNA) building. And lastly, ACoA is the raw material for making *cholesterol* and *long-chain fatty acids* (which form *triglycerides*).

ACoA, therefore, can become pretty-much anything, ranging from fuel to structural protein to artery-clogging cholesterol. Now, most healthy adults, who aren't growing like children do, or healing from, say, a major injury, or surgery, don't have much need for new proteins or new nucleic acids. What they do need is energy, but if they don't need energy at that very moment, when ACoA arrives on the scene, there is only one other place for ACoA to go: *Fatty acid and cholesterol production.*

Glucose metabolism, to review, hits a roadblock at the PFK reaction and only proceeds to ACoA if there is a need for energy or building blocks. If there is no such need, glucose gets stored as glycogen, which gets burned up *first* every time muscles do even a little work, or if the liver senses a dip in blood sugar. In short, when glucose is the simple sugar being burned, only enough ACoA gets produced to meet immediate needs.

But when fructose is the simple sugar, ACoA is generated with no regard for actual needs, and whatever isn't needed for fuel is mostly shunted off to fatty acid and cholesterol production. Blood triglycerides are elevated (200% higher after combined fructose-glucose ingestion, compared to pure glucose), and obesity is promoted by the deposition of excess triglycerides in adipose tissue throughout the body.

The Dark Side of the Force...I Mean, Fructose

Besides adversely impacting lipids and obesity, fructose fails to stimulate the release of insulin from the pancreas, leptin from fat, and GLP-1 from the small intestine. All three of these hormones are anorexigens, that is, they suppress the brain's appetite centers, and decrease feeding. Another way fructose hobbles appetite control is by failing to suppress *ghrelin*, which is the only circulating gut hormone that is an *orexigen*, that is, a substance that increases feeding. By failing to stimulate anorexigenic signals and suppress orexigenic ones, diets high in fructose increase energy intake, decrease energy expenditure, and favor weight gain. Or, as a 2005 article in *Diabetes Health* put it, increased fatty acid synthesis coupled with failure to properly regulate appetite-controlling hormones, "is like opening the flood gates of fat deposition." Furthermore, functional brain images following glucose versus fructose ingestion show that glucose reduces activity in those hedonic, or pleasure-seeking brain centers we talked about in Chapter 12, while fructose has no effect on them.

In other words, fructose fails to satisfy.

And, those biosynthetic building blocks ACoA can feed into producing…

Some of them are purines, which breakdown to uric acid, which can cause painful gout and kidney stones. Uric acid levels are higher in studies of fructose consumption, which have also linked fructose, but not glucose, with higher blood triglycerides, glucose, and LDL cholesterol, more abdominal fat, and greater insulin resistance.

In the National Health and Nutrition Examination Survey (NHANES 2003-2006) consumption of more than two-and-a-half HFCS-sweetened soft drinks per day was associated with a 77% greater risk of hypertension. There is also concern about fructose and nonalcoholic fatty liver disease, in which the liver becomes infiltrated with fat, leading to hepatitis and cirrhosis. The conversion of fructose to fatty acids inside the liver is the source of that concern, and a Duke University study links greater than seven fructose-sweetened beverages per week to fibrosis ("scarring") of the liver. Sadly, fatty liver disease is now the most common liver malady in children, affecting one-third of overweight kids.

According to researchers at the University of Oxford and the University of Southern California, countries that use HFCS in their food supply have a 20 percent greater prevalence of type 2 diabetes. Remarkably, between the HFCS countries and the non-HFCS countries, there were no differences in BMI, total calorie intake, and total sugar intake. One of the researchers, Michael I. Goran, PhD, stated HFCS "appears to pose a serious public health problem on a global scale…[and] may result in negative health consequences distinct from and more deleterious than natural sugar."

Noted Louisiana State University obesity expert, Dr. George Bray, recently addressed in *Diabetes Care* "whether there is a threshold below which fructose is without harm." He concluded there was not, that the problems with fructose have been a modest, natural aspect of human nutrition "for eons." He went on: "The reason we are now detecting the pathophysiological consequences of fructose is that its dietary load has continued to increase, largely as a consequence of increased soft drink and fruit drink consumption."

THE TRUTH IS, AS USUAL, IN THE MIDDLE

Astonishingly there remains debate as to the true health significance of HFCS. I recently read a point/counterpoint-type piece entitled: "Is High-Fructose Corn Syrup to Blame for Obesity in the United States?" And I have to say it was almost absurdly difficult to tell the two sides of the argument apart. It all boiled down to sugar being bad, and since HFCS is a lot of the sugar out there, HFCS is bad too. The "pro-HFCS" guy simply added the quite reasonable and correct point that HFCS is not the only factor driving the obesity epidemic, and eliminating it, or any "*one*" food, nutrient or ingredient," would not solve the obesity crisis.

My personal belief is that, while everything discussed above impacts the health of Americans, we have to recognize that fructose was around, naturally, in abundance, in our diets before HFCS was ever a gleam in some food scientist's eye. The small percentage increase in fructose intake resulting from the taste-equivalent substitution of HFCS for cane sugar might have had some direct consequences, but they might have been minimal, had not the absolute number of sugar calories consumed increased so dramatically—an increase HFCS certainly had a hand in.

But that's like blaming a gun for the guy pulling its trigger and killing another guy. HFCS isn't in and of itself poison; our misuse of it has made it poison. One of my pharmacology professors in medical school said all drugs were poison, just a matter of dose, turning something helpful, into something harmful. That's the case here. We have over consumed HFCS, and other sugars, to the point they are poisoning us.

Why and how have we done this?

Three synergistic explanations:

Economic

The lower cost and physical attributes of HFCS allowed the food and beverage industries to produce and market sugary products in great variety, packaged in large quantities, and to sell them at value prices. Human nature being what it is, presented with gobs of tasty calories, our habits changed to the point of overindulgence becoming the "new normal." What about countries that don't permit the use of HFCS? They have as much obesity as we do. That is yet another economic effect of HFCS. It drove the price of cane sugar down. Thus, manufacturers in countries without HFCS still "benefited" from lower sweetener costs, and so they too got to flood their consumer markets with the same excess of sweet foods and beverages as the HFCS countries.

Physiologic

The lack of effect of fructose on insulin, leptin, GLP-1, and ghrelin—hormones involved in energy balance—and hedonic brain activity, increases appetite and promotes over-consumption of all food categories: carbohydrates, fats, and proteins.

Misguided Public Education

The federal government and healthcare, with the cooperation of food-industry ingenuity and marketing, have for decades pushed a "low-fat" agenda—*low fat* being another way of saying *high carb*, and in this day and age, high carb almost unavoidably means HFCS rich.

THE SOLUTION?

As much as it surprises me to say, the solution is not to ban HFCS, even if that were likely. The solution is the same as it's been from page one:

Personal choice, personal empowerment.

Eat fewer calories.

Of all types.

Especially sugar.

Of all types.

Not just HFCS.

Now—do I think eliminating or significantly reducing HFCS (as I have done) is a good strategy for achieving that reduce-sugar-of-all-types goal?

Absolutely. A product with HFCS listed as a major ingredient is bound to be high in sugar. Just don't fool yourself that HFCS is the only culprit in the obesity epidemic. Also, before HFCS hijacked the discussion, recall that I was espousing "quality not quantity." HFCS, even if not inherently evil, has been a major tool of the quantity-not-quality bandwagon. I think it's fair to say that HFCS showing up fairly high on any ingredients list is a red flag for a lower quality product—that is, more processed, less natural. Dr. Goran, of the University of Southern California, whom I quoted above, stated in a separate interview: "It comes back to the need for a shift in social norms that will promote real foods and avoid processed foods, especially foods and beverages made with high-fructose corn syrup and reducing our cultural obsession with sugar and sweet taste."

Mary Franz, Harvard dietitian and respected authority on nutrition for diabetes, has offered the following tips on reducing sugar in general, which we should all do, regardless of whether one has diabetes:

- Scale back or eliminate non-diet soda, energy drinks, and sports drinks.*
- Check ingredients lists for all types of sugar, including HFCS; if more than two or three appear, especially if high on the list, put it back on the shelf. Other "sugar words": sucrose, dextrose, maltose, xylose, invert sugar, honey, molasses, fruit-juice concentrate, maltodextrin, turbinado sugar, malt syrup, brown rice syrup, and agave nectar.
- Buy 100 percent fruit juice and keep servings small.†
- Cut sugar in baking and cooking, using a half to a third less than the recipe calls for.
- Skip or share dessert

---

* I reproduced this list as Ms. Franz published it—but remember, it is not clear that "diet" drinks are really okay.

† My suggestion, not Ms. Franz's, but you might dilute juice in water or seltzer, producing a lower-calorie beverage, and in the case of the seltzer dilution, mimic the fizz of soda if that's something you miss.

16

NO SUCH THING AS A FREE LUNCH

The point of this chapter's title is to say there is no substitute for hard work and discipline, no easy way out, if you want to accomplish something meaningful—like earning a tough academic degree, or writing a great novel, or raising good kids…or achieving and maintaining a healthy BMI.

"SUGAR FREE"

A example of trying to take "the easy way out" has been discussed regarding diet sodas, and other uses of non-calorie sweeteners. It's not clear, as I've said, that the massive consumption and availability of non-caloric sweeteners and "sugar-free" products has helped the epidemic of obesity. Certainly, judicious use of these products as part of a larger, deliberate lifestyle that limits consumption of calories of all types, may not be unreasonable. What I am definitively advising against is the blind, haphazard substitution of Diet Pepsi for Pepsi, Equal for table sugar, Splenda in cake recipes, and so forth, without any thought to other calorie intake. You cannot latch onto any one tool, especially one provided by the same food industry that ushered us into the trouble we're in, and expect that one thing to solve all your problems. There must be other input, other effort, from you.

No such thing as a free lunch, or easy weight loss.

I closed the last chapter with a list of suggestions from Harvard dietitian Mary Franz, which included one to cut the amount of sugar called for in, for example, a cake recipe.

That's one approach to the particular problem of cakes and other baked goods, and I would prefer that to the substitute-Splenda approach, given the uncertainties as to the true efficacy of non-caloric sweeteners in combating obesity. But to expand upon this whole cutting/substituting notion—it is in some respects an "easy way out." Do it, every little bit helps (so long as it doesn't make the recipe truly inedible). But I'd really rather you put as much or more effort into training yourself to simply eat less cake.

It's harder to eat less cake than it is to change one ingredient, but eating less cake is more likely to get you to your goal. It helps you establish a habit applicable to all cakes you encounter (all foods in general, for that matter), not just ones whose ingredients you have total control over. Same with sugar-free bread. Better to eat less bread, period.

Why isn't it enough to just take the sugar out when baking? Because the wheat flour in bread and cake breaks down to glucose when eaten. In other words, plenty of sugar is being consumed even if nary an iota of granulated sugar is ever added. Now, to state the obvious, a cup of sugar has more sugar than a cup of flour—twice as much, in fact. Nevertheless, one measured cup of white all-purpose wheat flour contains 370 calories in the form of glucose. People who eat cake made with Splenda or using a reduced-sugar recipe, may be eating fewer carb calories than they would have, but they're eating a lot of carbs all the same, and if they aren't seriously accounting for that, they really shouldn't bother.

Another Tricky Marketing Ploy

The other day I saw in my office a middle-aged woman with diabetes, mystified why her blood sugars were out of control, because she was eating "right." When I asked for an example of what she was doing right—when I ask questions like this almost invariably the explanation is in the first words out of the patient's mouth—she reported was eating only sugar-free bread. It was news to her that there were still lots of carbohydrate calories in the flour the bread was made from. (Her husband sat rather smugly beside her saying, "I told you so.") This is another marketing danger zone. We've talked about *value for the money, supersizing, two for one*.

Sugar free is just another lure.

The food industry knows people are concerned about weight, and that labeling like "sugar free" or "fat free," when they can plausibly be applied, will encourage BMI-conscious shoppers to buy those products. Those labels, those products, like sugar-free bread, are there not because anybody has proven they do any good, not because the food industry cares about your health; they are there because they know *you* care about your health and will, they hope, buy into their marketing, growing their profits. It's not altruism, it's free enterprise, greed if you will. I don't wholeheartedly fault an effort to boost sales by setting one product apart from another, but I do fault the consumer for falling for it. We have to be smarter and we cannot be led around by the nose by the food industry. They do not have our best interests at heart, and we are fools to suppose that they do.

Even if there is a truly healthful motive behind the creation of some product, I still urge caution. Which "healthy-eating product" is real and which is hype? Think you can tell? Even if you can, and the product was honestly produced for the right reasons, in the right manner, or at least the manner intended, there is still a chance it is "misguided." Do we know the well-intentioned nutritional principle the product supports is really correct? If a food is stamped LOW FAT, should you grab it? Will you be the healthier for it?

Recall the disaster that was, in my opinion, the original food pyramid. In Chapter 8, I introduced Boston University obesity researcher Barbara Corkey. Dr. Corkey wrote in her *Diabetes Care* paper: "…the prevalent focus on the evils of dietary fat and their implied causative role in obesity are not well documented by scientific evidence. Indeed, the decrease in fat consumption that has resulted from abundant (nonevidence-based) medical and government advice against fat consumption has not decreased the burden of metabolic disease in our society."

Or as Dr. David L. Katz, Yale obesity expert, wrote in *Endocrine Today*: "We cut fat and got fatter and sicker…"

Yet, think how many products are on your grocer's shelves labeled to emphasize their lower-fat content. Better to do your own research, think out your own diet, make choices based on that. Do not buy something solely because it is stamped with a simpleminded label like "sugar free" or "fat free," anymore than you should buy something solely because of a two-for-one deal.

Success isn't in the Math

As I've said before, I think behavior and engraining good habits is more important to managing BMI, than arithmetic. The Splenda-laced/reduced-sugar-cake scenario is an example of this principle.

No doubt the person baking their cake with Splenda instead of sugar—all other things being equal—ends up with a lower-calorie cake, and the math would say eating that cake is healthier. But substituting Splenda just confuses things. People think Splenda-sweetened cake is a free food when it isn't. Even if they realize there are other calories in there, including lots of other carbs, there is a great danger of overeating, losing track. There is too much for us to juggle—what we're eating, how much we're eating, what we should eat more of and less of, other distractions like that big meeting, a crisis at home—and there is plenty of physiology driving us to eat more than intended, if we let our guard down, even just a little.

I say, keep it simple.

Stay focused, primarily, on how much you're eating, no matter what it happens to be. Sure, pay attention to ingredients and make better, higher-quality food choices, as we have extensively discussed. Once you've selected something for eating, however, no matter how "healthy" or "right" you think it is, focus on eating smaller servings.

With respect to the cake example, no matter how or how much you choose to sweeten your cake, eat less cake. Make cake less often. When you do have cake, cut smaller pieces, and don't eat the whole cake! Give away some, or freeze some, or—horror of horrors—throw it away. It may be a sin to waste food, but in our era, our society, gluttony is our greater sin. The garbage can is a healthier alternative to feeling obligated to eat it because it's there. If you can't live with throwing something away, don't buy it or make it, or else find somebody to finish it for you.

Oh, and before we leave this there's-no-easy-way-out topic, another example is the principle, discussed previously, but it bears reiterating, that it is not sufficient to focus on any single parameter in isolation. Improving food quality, for example, does not obviate our need to cut portions. We need to do both, and more.

17

BEYOND LIFESTYLE: DRUGS & SURGERY

Thus far we have dealt with just the first step in the overall treatment strategy for obesity as it exists today: namely, *self-directed lifestyle change*. "Self-directed" meaning, things you can do for yourself. Cutting portions. Modifying food and beverage choices. Getting more sleep. Exercising, both endurance and resistance. Only two aspects of weight management we've covered to this point are not self directed—the first being diseases that impact weight, like diabetes and hypothyroidism, thoughtful treatment of which require a physician's input. I emphasize *thoughtful*, because all-to-commonplace mismanagement of these conditions can completely sabotage one's weight-control efforts.

Second, are the weight-promoting drugs discussed in Chapter 8. Obviously it requires working with the prescribing provider to get off a drug that might be worsening a weight problem, and finding, if necessary, an acceptable alternative.

Following self-directed lifestyle change, assuming that fails to achieve ones weight-related goals, the next phase in the overall treatment strategy, as conceived by obesity-medicine specialists, is *professionally-directed lifestyle change*. This is the same as above, except with professional help: working with a dietitian, a health coach, a personal trainer; enrolling in a commercial weight-loss program like Weight Watchers; many YMCAs offer an intensive lifestyle modification program based upon the large Diabetes Prevention Program medical study.

The third and fourth phases in the progression of modern obesity therapy are, respectively, *adding medications* and *weight-loss surgery*. I'm going to discuss these in reverse order, although surgery is reserved—I don't want to say, "last resort," because in the right patient modern weight-loss surgery has a lot going for it—but, for obvious reasons, which include cost, surgery is generally reserved for those patients who are worst off, with the worst complications.

Nowhere is the heterogeneous nature of obesity, and the multimodal and individualized nature of successful obesity treatment, more important to understand, than when we start looking at these "add-on" therapies. And add-on therapies they are; weight-loss drugs and weight-loss surgery are not substitutes for, but rather additions to lifestyle change.

Make no mistake, not even surgery works for everybody, and without ongoing disciplined effort to maintain healthy lifestyle changes in the post-operative period, it will fail. It is very possible to out eat the restrictions placed on the GI tract by the various procedures, and regain the weight. I had a man in my office just the other day, who had a "Lap-Band" in place, and he told me his technique for eating whatever he wanted despite the reduced capacity of his stomach.

Wow! If anything ever opened my eyes to the need for a multidisciplinary approach, that no single intervention is ever likely to be the answer, that obesity is complex—it was that scene in my office. A man with an invasive device in place, who had paid a surgeon handsomely to place it, who had figured out a way to subvert the device, and gain his weight back. Do not misunderstand. I neither ridicule nor condemn this man; I am marveling at what we're up against. The power of the human brain—conscious and subconscious—to defend its set-point weight is simply stunning.

As we talk about moving beyond lifestyle changes to drugs and surgery, I admit two things: (1) I harbor a lot of compassion for, and share the frustration of, persons who are *morbidly* (that is, *severely* and *detrimentally*) obese. They have a big hole to dig their way out of, just using that hard work and discipline I'm touting, and it's harder for them to add physical activity to the equation, especially if serious orthopedic issues have developed. And (2) my comments about drugs and surgery for managing BMI will be relatively brief, and in contrast to the rest of this book, more based upon third-party references, less on my personal clinical experiences. Because, frankly, I've not used weight-loss drugs much in my career, and my direct involvement with weight-loss surgeries is, to date, almost nil.

Ask any mainstream endocrinologist or internist, and I'll bet nine times out of ten their reported experience will be similar to mine, especially with respect to medications. The epidemic of obesity and diabetes, though, is bringing on a kind of renaissance in obesity medicine—a rapid increase in interest in, and knowledge and experience about, non-lifestyle weight-loss therapies amongst rank-and-file doctors.

SURGERY

What I do have to say about *bariatric* (literally meaning, "weight-treatment") *surgery* is largely positive. Long-term follow up, over say ten years, of the severely obese shows very limited success with diets, behavioral therapies, exercise programs, and drug treatments. Nearly all patients regain whatever they lose. I recently saw a patient for her annual thyroid appointment. The prior year we had documented a one-hundred-pound weight loss compared to the year before that. She had used a commercial medically assisted weight loss program involving lifestyle counseling and appetite suppressants. At the latest appointment, though, we documented a one-hundred-pound *weight gain*. She gained it all back. "Surgery is currently the best-established...most successful method for sustained weight loss in the morbidly obese," according to a 2008 *Endocrinology and Metabolism Clinics of North America*.

Since the advent of bariatric surgery in the 1960s, much has been learned about preventing unacceptable complications (including liver and kidney failure, and severe vitamin and mineral deficiencies) that led to over 30,000 operations having to be undone in those early days, and modern laparoscopic techniques have transformed this field of surgery into one viewed as less invasive, and more acceptable in the eyes of both the public and physicians.

The safest, most effective procedure, and the one most commonly performed today is the *Roux-en-Y gastric bypass* (RYGB), usually done through a scope, without a major abdominal incision. The stomach is reduced to a pouch the size of a golf ball, and the small intestine is cut twelve inches beyond the duodenum, the far end pulled up and attached to the tiny stomach. This restricts calorie intake (the small stomach) and causes the malabsorption of those calories that do get through (the shortened bowel). In addition, there are alterations in gut and other appetite-modulating hormones and signals, such as ghrelin, GLP-1, and amylin, resulting from this rerouting, that actually improve, for example, diabetes within days, well in advance of significant weight loss.

In other words, contrary to common sense and conventional thought, the major benefit of RYGB seems to be physiological rather than mechanical—altered gastrointestinal signals to the brain, pancreas, and liver, dramatic effects on hunger and satiety, and an increase in basal metabolism. And that set point we've been talking about is readjusted downward, such that the brain defends a lower weight. But, it will defend that weight. Surgical patients lose down to the new set point then stabilize and lose no more. Very few patients become underweight after surgery.

Also, as already detailed in Chapter 9, RYGB changes the gut microbiota, the intestinal bacteria, to a profile more beneficial to weight loss. A feature of the surgery that seems important in this, which hasn't yet been mentioned, is that the free piece consisting of the rest of the stomach—severed from the esophagus—and the duodenum and upper small intestine are sewn into the lower intestine so that bile from the liver and gall bladder, emptying into the duodenum, passes into the lower intestine without previously having come in contact with food, which took the other pathway. This exposes lower intestinal bacteria to undigested food, altering the microbiota. This observation and others is leading to new technologies that may reproduce some of the key effects of RYGB, without having to perform a major operation. For example, a tube-like device placed in the GI tract that separates bile acids from one's ingested meal until the lower small bowel is reached.

Since 2001, *laparoscopic adjustable gastric banding ("The Lap-Band")* has become quite popular, but is falling out of favor. Its placement is a shorter operation than RYGB, but results in restriction only, not malabsorption, and effects on appetite-regulating hormones are lacking. Banding fails to drop the BMI to under 35 in over a third of cases, over five years, while only 4 percent of RYGBs fail that standard. RYGB produces greater weight loss and greater improvements in obesity-related diseases. There are other procedures, which I won't detail; however, none have uniformly improved upon RYGB.

Bariatric surgery, today, is among the safest of surgeries, remarkable considering obese patients tend to have more surgical complications in general. Nevertheless, complications do occur, including deaths, even with the Lap-Band. More deaths in fact occur after discharge than during hospitalization, a fact not fully understood. Severe nutritional deficiencies occur, as does life-threatening hypoglycemia (low blood sugar), perhaps as long as fourteen years postop. I mention these negatives to illustrate that, while I do believe bariatric surgery to be the best option for the very-obese, particularly those with diabetes and other obesity-related diseases, it is still not a solution to be taken lightly. It is certainly not an "easy out." Frankly, I think the prospect of bariatric surgery should scare the bejeezus out of anyone not yet at the point of no return, into redoubling their lifestyle efforts.

DRUGS

That brings us to my other category of non-lifestyle obesity treatment:

The proverbial "diet pill."

And just as the thoughtless application of non-caloric sweeteners, without addressing other issues is doomed to failure, so too is the thoughtless use of "diet pills"—better referred to as anti-obesity drugs, or *anorectics* (appetite-suppressants), although not all potential agents for obesity attack the appetite. Some decrease appetite, that is, reduce energy intake, and others increase energy expenditure, an example of the latter being thyroid hormone, a metabolic stimulator, which was the first deployed weight-loss drug, in 1893.

It was a disaster.

It caused life-threatening *thyrotoxicosis*—hyperthyroidism—and in the almost century-and-a-quarter since, many drugs tried on obesity have had to be removed from the market due to bad outcomes. Certainly, the reputation of obesity drug treatments has been tarnished over the years by their frequent chemical relationship to drugs of abuse ("speed"), marking many doctors prescribing them as "disreputable" (often they were), and by frequent toxicity problems, as follows:

1933	Dinitrophenol	Cataracts, nerve damage
1937	Amphetamine	Drug addiction
1967	"Rainbow" pills	Deaths*
1971	Aminorex	Pulmonary hypertension
1997	Redux, Fen-Phen	Heart valve erosion
2010	Meridia	Heart attack, stroke, death

---

* "Rainbow" referred to the horrid conglomeration (amphetamines, barbiturates, thyroid hormone, digitalis, diuretics, laxatives) given to patients by a proliferation of "fat doctors" in the 1960s, triggering a rash of deaths and a congressional investigation. The 1/26/68 *Life* magazine cover touted, "The Dangerous Diet Pills: How millions of women are risking their health…'"

Nevertheless, the obesity epidemic has reenergized skittish United States FDA regulators, who after a spate of disapprovals, approved two new products in 2012, for prolonged use against medically significant obesity, *Belviq* and *Qsymia*. Experience with these agents, to date, is limited. In fact, Belviq (generic name, locaserin) has only barely reached pharmacies at the time of this writing. These two agents join one surviving FDA-approved anti-obesity drug for long-term use: *orlistat*, the over-the-counter drug, *Alli*.

Compared to all other drugs for obesity, past and present, orlistat is a beacon of safety, and actually has proved to prevent diabetes. Use of it is limited, however, owing to unpleasant, though non-life-threatening side effects, including excessive flatulence (farting) and "explosive" diarrhea. Orlistat causes malabsorption of fat by the small intestine, and therefore is tolerable only if dietary fat is restricted. I have always thought of it as *Antabuse for fat*—Antabuse being an old drug, now fallen out of favor, that treats alcoholism by making the alcoholic sick when imbibing. The patient on orlistat is encouraged to eat relatively more carbohydrate calories, which concerns me as not being good for established diabetics, which is why I've stayed away.

A number of drugs are used off-label for obesity. These include certain antidepressants and antiepileptic drugs (bupropion, topiramate, and zonisamide) but most promising, to my thinking, are a selection of antidiabetic drugs with weight loss as one of their beneficial effects.

Metformin, with its weak weight-loss effect, is the oldest of these, and the only one dosed by mouth. *Byetta*, *Victoza*, and *Bydureon* are related drugs mimicking the GLP-1 gut hormone. These have a more robust effect on weight than metformin, but must be injected (twice daily, once daily, and weekly, respectively). They are also expensive. Another potential antidiabetic/weight-loss shot, *Symlin*, works slightly differently from the GLP-1 mimics, and is injected before each meal. It is also expensive. Cost is especially concerning for all these products—except generic metformin, which is dirt cheap—since insurance coverage for off-label use in non-diabetics will be iffy. (Hopefully the American Medical Association's recent declaration of obesity as a disease will loosen insurance purse strings.) These drugs, though, are obvious good choices for blood-sugar control in type 2 diabetics who are also obese. My experience is extensive using all these five in that setting, and I have to say the weight loss I've seen is very hit and miss, although it can occasionally be impressive.

Which bolsters the critical point that no one intervention, certainly no seeming quick-fix drug, is going to be *the* single answer to obesity. And just as there is no one-size-fits-all diet, different drugs will work differently on different people. In fact, among the principles of drug therapy adhered to by legitimate obesity-medicine specialists, yet often not by other prescribers of "diet pills," is to consider and give trials of multiple different drugs, selected based on the characteristics of each patient, until the one most effective and tolerable for that person is found. Also, rather than pushing one drug to the point of uncomfortable or risky side effects to get the desired weight loss, the experts use lower doses, that are more tolerable, and add a second drug, also at a low dose, once weight loss levels off on the first agent. In fact, the new drug Qsymia is a combination of low-dose *phentermine*—an amphetamine-like drug long used in obesity treatment—and low-dose, extended-release topiramate, one of those antiepileptic drugs used off-label for obesity.

There are four anorectics approved by the FDA for less than twelve weeks use—limited by safety concerns, including rapid heartbeat, and hypertension. The best known of these is *phentermine*, mentioned in the last paragraph. To date, I have rarely personally prescribed these agents because of the safety concerns, and because of my belief that any effective treatment of obesity would have to be of long duration. In fact, obesity specialists agree. One of their guiding principles being: *when drugs do work, they need to be continued long term, or else the benefit is lost*, the weight regained. (Which doesn't mean drugs don't work for obesity—after all, hypercholesterolemia and hypertension both return when their drugs are stopped too.)

Accordingly it is now commonly accepted medical practice to use phentermine, with proper precautions, for as long as is necessary, in other words, off-label use for longer than that specified twelve weeks.

Special Topics: One Thing I Do, Two I Refuse To

Thyroid. A word about thyroid hormone (e.g., *Synthroid, Armour Thyroid, Cytomel*) as obesity treatment. In most modern medical circles this is heresy. A dose of *levothyroxine* (generic Synthroid) given to a healthy person with normal thyroid function sufficient to cause weight loss will probably make the person hyperthyroid— hyperthyroidism being a serious disease we go to great pains to diagnose and treat when it occurs spontaneously.

That said, there has been rekindling of interest in this potential use of thyroid hormone in the endocrinology journals of late. There is work, for instance, seeking a *thyroid-hormone analogue* (a modified thyroid hormone) that produces weight loss without hyperthyroidism.

I don't suggest we give Synthroid or the like to anybody with normal thyroid levels. However, I do think it can help with weight loss in those who also happen to need therapy for low thyroid levels, i.e., *hypothyroidism*. In fact, I believe hypothyroidism to be underdiagnosed; I believe the thyroid blood tests used to declare a person "normal" are often inaccurate, or misinterpreted. So, there may be people who are obese and hypothyroid, who have been incorrectly told they are not hypothyroid. These people might see some weight loss, from Synthroid, were they to be prescribed it. Thus, a little extra investigation, little thinking outside the box, might avail some obese patients (those with occult or otherwise missed hypothyroidism) of the weight benefits of thyroid hormone. This is a complex subject, full of pitfalls, covered in depth in my book, *The Thyroid Paradox: How to Get the Best Care for Hypothyroidism*.

Jumpstarts. A patient occasionally presses me to prescribe an anorectic to "jumpstart" her weight-loss efforts. Reasonable, on its face, although I have always refused them. These drugs are mostly controlled substances, demanding a circumspection and professionalism on the part of the physician greater than the average prescription—for reasons of safety and (probably-low) addiction potential, as well as prudent observance of federal and state rules and statutes regarding dispensing of controlled drugs: whether or not one agrees with those rules and statutes. In any case, these drugs, like all drugs, have side effects, some dangerous—some completely unexpected, like the Fen-Phen heart-valve debacle.

With respect to those side effects, part of practicing good, ethical medicine is not prescribing any drug, or other therapy, unless the likely benefit clearly outweighs the risk. And since long experience shows that "jumpstarting" with a drug virtually never produces sustained weight loss, and since these drugs have risks, it is almost never going to be the case that I could, in good conscience, say the benefit outweighs the risk.

Patients who are obese, suffering obesity-related diseases, who need medications, need them long term. A jumpstart is not sufficient, and patients who aren't so bad off should not be exposed to the risks. Besides, going on and off drugs is no different than yo-yo dieting, and likely would result in a creep upward of the hypothalamic BMI set point.

There is a neurochemical explanation, but in colloquial English, my take is: the only way to change lifestyle enough to maintain weight loss (i.e., to alter the set point) is to change those habits from the beginning. Use them to get the weight off, then ease back a little, into a maintenance phase. That process is easier said than done—if drugs are used as a crutch, just as if non-calorie sweeteners are used as a crutch, it's impossible. No where close to the necessary healthy habits ever get laid down, cemented in place, consciously nor subconsciously.

Treating Non-Obesity. Occasionally a non-obese, non-overweight woman (I don't recall it ever being a man) requests a weight-loss prescription. She simply wants to lose weight—not for medical reasons, for personal ones, and there is nothing wrong with that provided the goal is a healthy one, not a desire, for example, to be underweight.

But in my opinion, and that of any responsible physician, anorectic drugs should never be used in normal-weight persons, or those only minimally overweight with no significant associated disease. Never, ever. And I question the priorities, maturity, really of an individual who would ask, even beg to be put on a powerful risky drug, when there is no clear medical reason to do so. These drugs, all drugs—anything strong enough to help is strong enough to hurt—should be *feared*, not desired, or at least regarded with a great deal of respect for what they can do…

Both good…

And bad.

Late-Breaking News

As I was getting this book ready, an event occurred which has the potential to change the whole complexion of drug therapy for overweight and obesity, or at least physicians' attitudes towards it, which has often been negative, my own included. In May 2013, at their annual meeting in Phoenix, the American Association of Clinical Endocrinologists rolled out their "New Comprehensive Diabetes Management Algorithm," developed by a task force of nineteen top endocrinologists. It is a massive, complex document, most of which is beyond our scope.

The part I want to highlight is, first, that in each major section—on treating prediabetes, type 2 diabetes, and lipid disorders (e.g., high cholesterol)—they specifically call for *medically assisted weight loss* as part of lifestyle modifications. And in a separate section focusing on overweight and obesity, they call for the prescribing of anorectic drugs to those patients with a BMI greater than or equal to 27, who had any degree of complications, whether cardiometabolic (e.g., diabetes, heart disease) or biomechanical (e.g., arthritis, bad feet), who failed to lose sufficient weight via lifestyle changes, bolstered by, for example, physician or dietitian counseling. They specified four drugs to be considered: phentermine, orlistat, *Belviq*, and *Qsymia*.

This is a bold step for a major mainstream medical organization. I applaud it. It is a wake-up call, emphasizing that we (physicians and patients) need to be using every tool in our box to try to combat the epidemics of obesity and diabetes, which constitute a true public-health crisis. And if these drugs carry risks, or are imperfect—well, the same can be said, to one degree or another, of most drugs we prescribe. Therapeutic decisions always involve deciding which is worse, which is likely to do more harm—the cure, or the disease. In this case, the disease is doing a lot of harm, and should be, literally, treated as such.

It may even be if we move the anorectic drugs more into the offices of mainstream physicians—family practitioners, internists, endocrinologists, maybe cardiologists—and out of the "shadows" of the make-a-quick-buck, storefront weight-loss clinic, that we will learn to use them better, more safely and effectively. I'm enthusiastic about that prospect, either with the current crop of drugs, or those in the pipeline, like human recombinant leptin.

18

ONE DAY AT A TIME

C an a patient be addicted to food?

An *addiction* is a pathologically intense drive to consume a specific substance, or perform a certain behavior, not necessary for life. In the absence of that substance or behavior, uncomfortable symptoms appear, such as the physical illness resulting from narcotics withdrawal, or the intense seeking of the substance or behavior to the detriment of other areas of life (such as a gambling addict risking the family's finances, or a sex addict risking his marriage).

Most people who consume calories to the point of obesity are not "addicted" to food. They are succumbing to physiologically normal, healthy, robust appetites that conveyed a survival advantage in past times of frequent famines, but which is disadvantageous in our modern society of plenty.

I've just stated my own opinion, and that's the position this book takes on *food addiction*. To be sure, however, there is legitimate science, and debate about food addiction. And admittedly, in previous chapters I have made reference to the brain's hedonic, or pleasure/reward-seeking centers, and their role in the complex signals traveling between the gut and other organs, and the central nervous system, which regulate appetite and metabolism. These same hedonic centers, it turns out, are involved in the traditional addictions.

Thus, it may be relevant to consider something analogous to the traditional addictions as one of the numerous heterogeneous factors contributing to obesity. Some of the anorectic drugs discussed in the last chapter might well be, literally, treatments for food addiction. For example, one experimental drug combination for obesity, that has so far not passed FDA muster, is *naltrexone*, which includes an opioid blocker (heroin and morphine are examples of opioids, not to put too fine a point on this).

But, unless and until we get a practical, safe, affordable drug or drug combination to combat the addictive aspects of food, I believe *the notion of food addiction is best banished from our thinking*. It's not that I have my head in the sand about the science, but this is a practical book, presenting what I think to be practical techniques for weight loss today.

And with that in mind, does a diagnosis of food addiction help or hurt us?

To my thinking the vast majority of overweight or obese humans are not addicts—at least, they shouldn't be thought of or think of themselves as such. Food-seeking behavior is necessary for life. These people are instead suffering the consequences of normal neuroendocrine physiology thrust into a vat of abundance and marketing and poor nutritional education and poor nutritional science. To label a patient, allow a patient to go on labeling themselves, a "food addict" is harmful. It pastes a diagnosis on something physiologically normal.

It pastes an *excuse* on it.

If I am obese because I suffer food addiction, it isn't my fault. I am a victim of my disease. That might be comforting, but it doesn't solve the obesity problem. If, on the other hand, I accept that my weight issues developed against a background of normal physiology, then I am not a victim, I am not sick, I have control. That's an important psychological concept: if I have control, if the problem is at least partially my fault, then I have it in my power to fix said problem.

However—

I will for the purposes of this chapter use and embrace a phrase associated with the treatment of addictions.

Alcoholics Anonymous, and other twelve-step programs, have as one of their oft-quoted slogans: "One day at a time." The newly sober alcoholic facing that long trying road is counseled by his mentor to take it "one day at a time." I've already quoted radio financial counselor Dave Ramsey expressing a similar sentiment to callers facing huge debts: "How do you eat an elephant? One bite at a time."

In both situations the individual faces the daunting challenge of modifying entrenched behaviors, requiring self-discipline be brought to bear on numerous choices in any given day. The choice, in the case of the alcoholic, to take a shot of bourbon, or not; for the indebted to blow the monthly budget buying a new dress on impulse, or not; for the person trying to lose weight, to eat that Krispy-Kreme, or not...

I think it important to have timely feedback from our bodies about how we're doing, and to use that information when facing those choices throughout our days that impact our success. This brief chapter presents a simple technique I developed in the course of my own efforts that I suggest you try.

One day at a time.

WEIGH EVERY DAY?

I've heard advice that a person trying to lose weight should not weigh daily. There is a sound basis for that. There are day-to-day, hour-to-hour fluctuations, up and down, in body weight, due to many factors having nothing to do with stored fat calories. Such factors include hydration, salt intake, hormonal status, if you've recently consumed a large meal, when your last bowel movement was. Obviously clothing affects your weigh-ins, so I would take great care to make sure you're wearing about the same thing each time you weigh, or better yet, weigh at home without clothing.

Because of physiologically normal, unavoidable fluctuations, a more accurate assessment of one's overall progress can be obtained from, say, weekly checks, rather than daily ones. I thus agree with a no-more-than-once-a-week weigh-in, from the standpoint tracking progress.

On the other hand, there is value in weighing every day. Not for the purpose of tracking progress, but to provide a short-term reminder of what's at stake as you live each day making numerous food-and-beverage choices. Several published studies have, in fact, demonstrated greater reduction in BMI with daily self-weighing compared to, for example, weekly weigh-ins.

I suggest you weigh *every morning*, first thing, naked, right after voiding the bladder, using a good quality scale, preferably a digital one. I also recommend you have in mind, before weighing, a range, of say five pounds, you would consider acceptable for that day. The range takes into account the fluctuations mentioned above. Determining that range is easiest if you have already lost weight and are focusing on staying put. Just decide on a range that is acceptable to you, no less than two or three pounds above and below some average: say, 125–130 pounds.

If, however, you're still losing weight, the acceptable range will be a downward moving target bracketing some recent average. Say, your last "official" weigh-in was 180 pounds: if your goal is to lose a pound per week, then you want to end the present week with an average weight of about 179 pounds. Applying my give-or-take-two-or-three-pounds rule, your acceptable range this week will be, say, 176–182. The following week the acceptable range will frame-shift downward to, say, 175–181, the week after, 174–180, and so forth.

What do we do with these ranges?

With each morning check, compared to the current acceptable range, you will determine how aggressive you need to be with your calorie-restricting efforts that day. Again, the maintenance phase is easiest. If you're above your range, you need to be very strict that day: no desserts, no treats, maybe stick with salads and vegetables. Not that you shouldn't be leaning that way all the time, but for this one day you need to be extra careful. If you're within range, be careful but you can afford to be a little less strict, and if you're below the range—you're golden! Treat yourself a little, have a little fun, it's a free day—more or less.

If you are not in the maintenance phase, if you are still in the weight-losing phase, same guidelines, just a little more strict at each level. This is art, not science. But certainly, if you are trying to lose, and you are above the acceptable range that morning then that needs to be a very strict day, maybe even a day to skip a meal—one meal, not two, and never all.

Very important: *Do not panic about fluctuations within the acceptable range.* There are all kinds of good reasons for them. If the range this week is 176–182 pounds, and yesterday you were 177, and today you're 180, do not beat yourself up over it and do not act baffled in frustration by it. It's natural. In fact, a benefit of this technique is to illustrate, and educate, how much one's weight can vary from day to day. Just be very careful how you use the data you collect. If you are within range, whether up or down compared to the previous day— you are forbidden to worry about it.

And if you are fortunate enough to be down, remember:

Matter is neither created nor destroyed.

As a result of anything you ate or drank the previous day, you will not gain any more weight—in fact, that is true regardless of where your weight is, what direction it moved. Wherever you are in the morning, you are done with the previous day. You will not gain more because of anything you did, good or bad. The weight of the fat you will eventually store as a result of a previous single day's indiscretions cannot exceed the weight of what you swallowed. Every day is a new day. Each day starts fresh, with a different strategy, a different level of intensity to your weight-loss efforts, depending on that morning's weight.

I believe day-to-day, self-correction like this is far preferable to— and more flexible and enjoyable than—battling to maintain the same level of intensity and focus day in and day out over weeks and months, perhaps years.

19

GLYCEMIC INDEX: PARTS IS PARTS?

In simplest terms, *glycemic index* (GX) is a rank ordering of how high and fast a food spikes your blood sugar. Mathematically, GX is the ratio, expressed as a percentage, of the "glucose spike" of the test food, over the same subject's spike after consuming a standard meal of either white bread or glucose dissolved in water. Thus, the GX of white bread would be 100, as would be the GX of glucose water—illustrating, by the way a key point about carbohydrate consumption. White bread, or more basically, wheat flour, acts in the body no differently than sugar. One could therefore argue, from a health and nutrition perspective, if you wouldn't fill the palm of your hand with table sugar and slam it back, then you shouldn't eat white bread either. "Food" for thought.

Published GX tables reflect the average calculated from testing eight or ten volunteers. Often the terms *high-glycemic-index* and *low-glycemic-index* are incorrectly used as if interchangeable with, respectively, *high-carbohydrate* and *low-carbohydrate*. However, it is not only the carbohydrate content of a food that determines its GX. In fact, all foods tested are consumed by test subjects in amounts containing exactly fifty grams of carbohydrate, and are compared to fifty grams of carbohydrate from the white bread meal, or glucose water.

In other words, GX determinations deliberately exclude, or negate, consideration of the actual carbohydrate content of the food in question. GX is, therefore, not so much a *quantitative* measure of carb intake, but rather a *qualitative* measure. What is the quality, the metabolic nature of a particular episode of carbohydrate consumption.

Because it's calculation excludes consideration of actual carb content, GX may be misleading in certain real-world situations. Carrots, for example, a healthy food by most accounts, has a whopping GX of 131—a glucose spike 31 percent worse than white bread!

Except, nobody in their right mind, outside a nutrition lab, ever eats the one-and-a-half pounds of carrots necessary to get the fifty grams of carbohydrate that produces that 131 percent spike.

Another parameter, *glycemic load*, reformulates the GX into the context of realistic portion sizes. Glycemic load (GL) equals GX expressed as a ratio (131 becomes 1.31) multiplied by the number of carbohydrate grams consumed. Using published GX tables, anyone can plug in serving sizes (in grams carbohydrate), and determine the impact of and healthy-eating value of foods they're choosing from, vis-à-vis BMI- and diabetes-management.

Examples:

- One carrot (GX 131, 4 carb grams)—GL = 5 (1.31 x 4 = 5)
- One potato, mashed (GX 104, 37 grams)—GL = 38
- One cup of cooked pasta (GX 71, 40 grams)—GL = 28

So, carrots are good, mashed potatoes are bad, pasta falls somewhere in the middle—all of which meets my common-sense test. So, what determines GX, if not carbohydrate content?

- *The swelling of microscopic starch granules by heat and water:* granules swollen to the bursting point in a baked potato are more easily digested, yielding a higher GX, than unswollen ones in brown rice.

- *Food processing:* wheat ground into superfine flour has a higher GX than coarsely ground wheat grains; flour has greater surface area for digestive attack, and lacks the tough fibrous coating of the whole grain.

- *Fiber content:* indigestible fiber shields digestible food, spreading out release of sugars to the circulation.

- *Fat content:* fat consumed as part of the same meal (butter and sour cream on a baked potato, or a fatty piece of meat eaten with the same potato) slows the emptying of the stomach into the small intestine, where absorption occurs.

One might conclude the less cooked, less processed a food is, the more healthy it is, with respect to GX. This is by no means the whole healthy-eating story; however, it lends support to the "raw-food" movement, and the consuming of more "natural" or "whole" foods.

Let's be clear, though—neither glycemic index nor glycemic load should be the sole determiner of whether to include a food in one's meal plan. Eliminating carbohydrate-rich foods also eliminates the brain's major fuel source, as well as a lot of valuable fiber, vitamins, and minerals. If there is a range of acceptable choices, the serving with the lowest GL is probably the better pick. Just be cautious about popular diets built totally around low-GX eating. Just as in politics, it's dangerous to focus too much on one issue dogmatically, to the exclusion of all others.

The quintessential low-GX diet is the Atkins program, popularized in the early 1970s. Other examples include plans detailed in *Sugar Busters!* and *The South Beach Diet.* I recommend both books to my patients, but it is with the caveat that they use the information about the presumed benefits of low-GX eating, and the data in their GX tables, to help construct a diet, of their own, that works for them, is palatable to them. In other words, they should educate themselves, think for themselves, not robotically follow any one guru's spiel.

WHY LOWER GLYCEMIC LOAD?

If matter and energy are neither created nor destroyed, why care how rapidly the carbohydrate portion of a meal is absorbed? It's all going to the same place, right? Same number of calories consumed, absorbed, metabolized—into work, body-heat generation, storage as glycogen or fat—regardless of how fast they get digested, right? Isn't a calorie equal to a calorie equal to a calorie?

Parts is parts!

That argument is correct as far as it goes, but it oversimplifies human physiology. It focuses on math, not on behavior, not on the physiology and pathophysiology that influence behavior. Those gut-brain signal pathways for instance. And conquering obesity is at least as much about behavior as mathematics, about fooling those signal pathways.

There are three reasons to be concerned about big glucose spikes triggered by high-glycemic-load ingestions. One of those reasons relates solely to blood-sugar control in diabetics; the other two relate to weight management in general, diabetics and nondiabetics alike.

First, in a diabetic, I take it as obvious that, all other things being equal, a lower glycemic load will yield a lower after-meal blood glucose. A higher glycemic load will, on the other hand, produce a higher blood sugar, and if consumed regularly, will cause poorer overall blood-sugar control, and an increased risk for diabetes complications.

The remaining two benefits, more universal benefits, of a focus on GX, both involve insulin: the effect of post-meal glucose levels on insulin release, and insulin's subsequent impact.

The Insulin Factor

Glucose spikes begat insulin spikes, and *insulin is the fat-storage hormone.* It is the body's traffic cop directing calories toward that big parking garage known as adipose tissue, body fat. The more insulin a person is exposed to, the heavier he or she is likely to be. Supporting this theory is a compelling study published in a 2012 edition of *Cell Metabolism.* Mice with higher insulin levels were compared with mice genetically engineered to be incapable of making large amounts of insulin. The low-insulin mice did not gain weight on a high-fat diet. Their energy expenditure was, in fact, higher. Their calorie-storing white fat seemed to be converted to calorie-burning brown fat.

So, the first issue favoring a low-GX diet for weight loss is the metabolic promotion of fat storage by insulin.

The second relates to the more immediate, better known effect of insulin—blood-glucose lowering, more specifically, glucose transport across cell membranes out of blood capillaries, out of the blood.

Glucose spikes begat insulin spikes, which begat glucose plunges. A rapidly rising glucose may be followed quickly by a rapidly falling glucose. *And our bodies hate rapidly falling glucoses. With a passion.* They trigger an urgent physiologic response, which insists upon, via uncomfortable symptoms, an urgent response from the individual. When those symptoms are severe and come to medical attention, we call that *reactive hypoglycemia.*

More to say shortly about reactive hypoglycemia; it gets its own chapter, in fact. For now, suffice it to say, one of the symptoms of mild hypoglycemia, a dip in blood glucose, is hunger. When glucose spikes, insulin spikes, glucose drops, the person gets—hungry!

And when people get hungry, they eat.

High-GX eating leads to more rapid hunger, begetting more calorie intake, begetting weight gain and obesity. *Satiety* is what this boils down to: eat a low-GX diet and you're liable to feel more satiated, more full, for a longer time, wait longer before eating again, and ultimately you might consume fewer calories.

So, it is true, a calorie is a calorie is a calorie; a calorie (with apologies to Shakespeare) by any other name would pack as much metabolic energy. It is not that the total calories in any given meal have any different potential for *directly* impacting weight than an equal number of calories from a different meal. Rather, the advantage of lowering the glycemic load is *indirect*, related to future eating.

We're talking about modulating appetite—fooling our stomachs, altering those gut-brain signals. Five hundred high-GX calories will produce the same weight gain as 500 low-GX calories. The latter, however, will effect an appetite and behavioral change, lessening further calorie consumption across the rest of the day. This notion meshes perfectly with my advice to eat larger meals earlier, and perhaps just a small supper, or no supper. A sizable low-GX breakfast might satisfy to lunch with little or no snacking, and a similarly designed, medium-sized lunch, might do the same through the afternoon. By suppertime, the lowered glycemic load of the earlier meals will aid in curbing the evening appetite.

Eating any large meal at night, especially a low-GX one, should be infrequent. Remember, some of the benefit of lowering the glycemic load is that the meal remains in the stomach longer. I don't want a still-full stomach when I go to bed, which can incite, for example, acid reflux and heartburn.

Macronutrient Clarity

This is a good place to broaden the discussion of dietary macronutrient composition. The three *macronutrients* are fats, carbohydrates, and proteins. All nutritional strategies can be usefully categorized according to their relative macronutrient composition: high-fat, low-fat, high-carb, low-carb, high-protein, low-protein.

It's already been said that a low-GX diet is not necessarily the same thing as a low-carbohydrate diet. The glycemic index rather describes a quality particular to the carbohydrates that are chosen, regardless of the overall percentage of total calories made up by those carbohydrates. You could have a relatively high-carb diet that was composed of mostly low-GI foods—certain plant-based, vegetarian diets could meet those criteria.

By the same token, another common misconception is that low-GI equals high-protein or high-fat. I've looked at several GX tables and haven't seen steak or eggs or lard listed. That's because there aren't any carbohydrates to speak of in those calorie sources, and so it is impossible to feed a test subject a serving of steak with 50 grams of carbohydrate, with which to compare glucose spikes with the white-bread 50-gram-carb serving.

Enough with being compulsively precise about the terminology and mathematics—there comes a time when we just need to be practical. And from a practical standpoint, everybody requires some balance of fats, carbohydrates, and proteins. There are particular situations, up to and including personal preferences, where it is desirable to weigh the percentages more heavily toward one macronutrient or another. If one is hoping to construct a diet that blunts glucose spikes for the purpose of improving diabetes control and/or managing weight, then some mix of lower-GX carbs, plus some variety of quality meats and fats, to include olive oil, is reasonable and practical. It is also reasonable and practical, though not strictly correct, to think of the purer protein and purer fat components of your diet as having a GX of zero.

Thus, without getting bogged down in the mathematics, I think a working knowledge of the concept of GX, and a passing familiarity with where certain foods fall on the GX tables, can lead one to the easy, practical conclusion that a meal consisting of rib eye steak, green beans, and a mixed green salad with oil and vinegar, will spike ones post-meal glucose less than a similar sized meal of spaghetti with meat sauce and garlic bread.

COMMON SENSE VERSUS DOGMA

The value of paying attention to the GX has long made sense to me, especially in diabetics. And there were observations as to the weight-reducing benefits of lower-carb/higher-fat dieting as far back as the 1930s, and farmers have long known the way to fatten livestock is to force-feed grains and corn.

Yet, until recently, low-GX diets were looked upon as quackery—worse, *dangerous* quackery—by many mainstream physicians. It baffles me why so many very smart doctors—smarter and better paid than me!—resisted this notion for so long. I remember, perhaps ten years ago, a top diabetologist arguing against my support of patients using the *Sugar Busters!* plan, saying, "They just can't maintain it over the long run." Well, I'd argue that to be a flaw in all nutritional therapies, not a reason to condemn one over another. Even today I see dietitians teaching relatively high carbohydrate ingestion in diabetics. It is not unusual, I'm sorry to say, to see patients come back from the dietitian with higher blood sugars than they started with. This harkens back to, I believe, a bygone era when all available antidiabetic therapies carried dangerous hypoglycemia (low blood sugar) as a side effect. We are now, however, approaching the third decade of diabetes therapies that do not promote hypoglycemia, and so-called analogue insulins, which, while they can cause it, are far safer than older products.

Thus, we can be more cavalier today about cutting calories and carbohydrates in all people, regardless of diabetes status, without risking low blood sugars. I think this explains some of the resistance that has existed over the years against low-GX diets—the past reality, and a lack of realization that that reality has changed. If a diabetes patient is on, say, insulin, or a pill that can cause hypoglycemia, and he cuts calories, and his blood sugar runs low, I would cut the insulin or pill dose, not increase the carbohydrate intake. There are nuances to treating diabetes we needn't detail here, but for the vast majority, it is counterproductive to increase calories just to take a drug safety, to avoid hypoglycemia. To do so simply promotes more obesity.

A Great Awakening

In recent years, I'm pleased to say, resistance from medical experts against low-GX diets has lessened. (And by the way, let me remind you, at this juncture: a good diabetic diet is a good diet for all.) The American Diabetes Association's *Standards of Medical Care in Diabetes– 2013*, state: "The mix of carbohydrate, protein, and fat may be adjusted to meet metabolic goals and individual preferences of the person with diabetes" and "for weight loss, either low-carbohydrate, low-fat...or Mediterranean diets maybe effective..." The same guidelines hold there to be "no most effective mix [of carbs, fats, and proteins] that applies broadly and...proportions should be individualized." And: "A variety of dietary meal patterns are likely effective in managing diabetes including Mediterranean-style [heavy on fruits, vegetables, fish, olive oil, nuts, and wine], plant-based...low-fat and lower-carbohydrate eating patterns."

Numerous studies have shown greater weight loss and better control of cholesterol and triglycerides with low-carbohydrate compared to low-fat diets, at least in the first few months. A 2004 study did show the weight benefit was lost at the one-year point— that is, by one year, the low-carb and low-fat groups had lost the same amount of weight; however, the low-carb group, at one-year, still had better triglycerides, HDL cholesterol, and glucose levels. A paper presented at the 2013 American Association of Clinical Endocrinologists meeting in Phoenix compared high-protein with high-carbohydrate diets. Despite similar amounts of weight loss, the high-protein diet was associated with impressive improvements in insulin resistance, insulin production, glucose and triglyceride levels, resting metabolic rate, and C-reactive protein (an inflammation marker for increased risk of heart attack and stroke).

Overall, these studies show that people on lower-carb diets in many respects do better, and at the very least, don't do worse. Of great interest, nonalcoholic fatty liver disease, present in 74 percent of obese subjects, improved to a greater degree with dietary carbohydrate restriction than with fat restriction, despite equal weight loss, illustrating a critical general point:

None of us should be making assumptions, seeming simple and obvious, with respect to complex metabolic issues. It seems simple and obvious that eating fat would cause more fatty liver damage than eating high-fructose corn syrup, or other carbohydrates, right? Yet the opposite is true.

It seems simple and obvious that blood triglyceride and LDL cholesterol levels would be worse on a high-fat diet than a high-carb diet, yet that has not always proved to be the case.

I believe the main reason low-GX diets were marginalized, viewed as quackery, for so long is because advocating for them was diametrically opposed to the fundamental public-health message of the last fifty years:

Right up there with *Don't smoke!*

Don't eat fat!

And low-fat is virtually the same as saying high-carb. And vice versa. A low-carb, or less-carb message, is the same as a more-fat message. And anybody saying *that* prior to…*maybe* 2004, was running headlong into about ten speeding locomotives. A phalanx of huge federal investments in public education, and physicians and nutritionists and other researchers whose careers were completely built on and invested in a *fat-is-bad* paradigm.

Let me not mince words:

This was a disaster.

We not only ignored benefits, or at least lack of harm, of low-GX dieting, for decades, but we drove people, insistently, hubristically, massively in the completely opposite direction. Causing, or at least exacerbating—as I've argued elsewhere—the epidemic of obesity we face today.

How did so many experts get it wrong?

A whole field of scientific endeavor?

Surely there were individual researchers with my same thoughts. Obviously Dr. Atkins, a graduate of Cornell University Medical College, and the three physician authors of *Sugar Busters!*, all graduates of respected US medical schools, were putting in a lot of relevant thought, years and decades before I knew enough to. Why did it take until less than ten years ago, as of this writing, for low-GX dieting to even start to be taken seriously?

I have some thoughts on that, the airing of which, at this point, would be an unforgivably digressive. Therefore, I have relegated them to this book's second appendix. The point being that the system by which interventions like low-GX dieting get scientifically evaluated and accepted or rejected is flawed. It is not an evil system, merely an imperfect one—as is all human endeavor.

Worse though than academic/research medicine's imperfections, is its refusal to see its flaws—and our (meaning community physicians') often blind, ring-in-the-nose following of it.

SELECTIVE USE OF THE GLYCEMIC INDEX IN WEIGHT MANAGEMENT

A book published in the late 1990s, *Eat Right For Your Type*, written by a naturopathic physician, has garnered much public notice. I am aware of no mainstream support for its premise that one's blood type (O, A, B, or AB, *that* blood type) determines, or is a marker for, what is the best diet for that individual, and to be clear, I do not endorse this book—although I admit when I got a copy and skimmed it, I did not find its notions and explanations nearly as quackish as I expected to.

At the very least I agree with its general proposition that the best nutritional plan for losing and maintaining weight is not the same for everybody. As I have said, human biology is diverse; it is folly to try to draw detailed conclusions that apply to everyone.

My version of "eat right for your type" involves *insulin resistance*. This metabolic derangement is thought to be caused by inherited genes that predispose to aggressive energy storage in the form of fat, as well as to the development of T2DM, and other diseases including polycystic ovary syndrome, hypertension, hyperlipidemia, acne, even heart disease and stroke. If you are diabetic, or have parents or siblings with diabetes, you are likely insulin resistant. If you have both parents with diabetes, you inherited more of those genes and your insulin resistance is probably worse. Insulin resistance, basically, means your body is not programmed to absorb and burn glucose easily and efficiently; carbohydrate ingestion causes higher glucose spikes, higher insulin spikes, more storage of calories as fat.

Thus, if you have type 2 diabetes, or a significant family history of it, I believe you should follow a low-GX/low-carbohydrate/higher-protein diet, and that such a diet will more readily result in weight loss, since insulin levels will be kept lower, and not tend to trigger as much expansion of fatty tissue, or excess between-meal snacking. Also the higher-protein component will build muscle, coupled with the resistance training advocated in an earlier chapter.

If you are not insulin resistant, perhaps simply cutting calories, carbs and fats equally, with less regard for the GX seems more reasonable. Higher protein intake though is probably helpful in all groups. Protein builds muscle, or prevents the loss of muscle that tends to occur with weight loss, and the more muscle you have, the more calories you burn both at rest and during exercise.

A 2005 paper out of Tufts University, Boston, supports my concept, reporting that a low-glycemic-load diet better facilitated weight loss in overweight adults with high insulin secretion (a marker for insulin resistance), than those with low insulin secretion.

For those lucky enough to not have a personal or family history of diabetes: you still might consider trying a low-GI diet as part of your exploration of various kinds of weight-loss diets, searching for the one that works best, and is most palatable. One theoretical benefit of a complete shift in macronutrient composition—like switching from low-fat to low-carb, or to a Mediterranean diet—is that such a shift might just be the shock you needed to lower your brain's set point for weight, which simple calorie cutting without a macronutrient shift might not readily do.

Practical Advice for Lowering Glycemic Load

Tables of foods ranked for GX can be found in any number of books on the subject, and no doubt all over the Internet. But you can also use common sense: take a food item—say, a piece of fruit, a whole apple—the more natural it is, the less processed it is, the lower its GX probably is. The more processed it is, easier it is to digest, the faster its carbohydrate calories are unleashed, the higher its GX probably is.

An apple is better than apple sauce is better than apple juice is better than apple juice concentrate. Another example: oatmeal. Steel-cut oats, rock-hard nuggets, have to be boiled twenty or thirty minutes to be edible, and are healthier than rolled oats, where the nuggets have been flattened, and cook faster, which are healthier than instant oatmeal which is treated to make the oats soften to the point of consumability by merely stirring in hot water.

The more processed, more convenient a food is, the less healthy it probably is, and the more likely it is to adversely impact your weight and blood sugar. Meals should be savored and toiled over. They are not meant to be cheap, nor easy, nor fast. I never eat instant oatmeal. If I have oatmeal, I boil steel-cut oats for a half-hour, stirring frequently and attentively.

No time for that? I completely understand—I don't have oatmeal that often, in fact—but I advise either finding the time, or not eating oatmeal, especially if you have diabetes or are struggling with obesity. This is a tiny example of how modern stressed, hurried, two-income-household lifestyles, necessitating the likes of instant oatmeal, has contributed to the epidemic of obesity.

20

REACTIVE HYPOGLYCEMIA

R*eactive hypoglycemia* is a lowering of blood sugar resulting from the post-meal insulin spike, to the point the patient feels uncomfortable, possibly with debilitating symptoms, which generally fall short, though, of the devastating effects of "true hypoglycemia" caused by, for example, overly aggressive diabetes therapy, or an insulin-secreting tumor. Such severe hypoglycemia can cause seizures, disorientation, sudden loss of consciousness, possibly causing a motor vehicle accident, if one is driving when the episode strikes. Again, it is important to note that patients with reactive hypoglycemia, a relatively common problem, almost never have events so severe. A reactive-type hypoglycemia, however, can occur and be quite serious in people following bariatric surgery and other surgeries interfering with absorption of calories from the gut.

I will limit my further comments to garden-variety reactive hypoglycemia in nonsurgical patients, typically young women. The story is a common one—this was a fad epidemic of the eighties—a young woman eats, perhaps unhealthily, high carbs, say a donut, washed down with a Pepsi. An hour or two later she feels weak, shaky, sweaty, her heart races, maybe she feels a sense of dread, she's hungry. These are early symptoms of a dip in blood sugar. They result from epinephrine (aka, adrenaline) release, which among other things stimulates glucose release from muscle and liver glycogen. Mobilizing these stores is physiologically normal and beneficial for the person whose blood sugar is dipping.

Our young, likely thin, though not always, female patient feels awful, having one of these spells she gets a couple hours after eating.

Someone suggests it sounds like hypoglycemia, low blood sugar, and gives her a Coke to drink, candy to eat. Within fifteen minutes she has completely recovered.

Except, the carbohydrates she ate and drank begat another insulin spike, which drops her blood sugar again. The symptoms are back, she thinks she's dying, doesn't know what is happening to her body, she is terrified, which releases—what?—epinephrine.

Adrenaline.

The fight-or-flight hormone.

The same stuff already pouring out as a result of the low blood sugar, or would be pouring out if Freddy Krueger were chasing her down the street with an axe. So, fear caused by the hypoglycemic symptoms, caused by epinephrine, triggers more epinephrine, more of the same symptoms.

A classic vicious cycle ensues:

> LOW BLOOD SUGAR ➜ SYMPTOMS ➜ FEAR ➜ MORE
> SYMPTOMS ➜ MORE FEAR

But by now she has learned that eating something sweet and drinking soda helps, and a second vicious cycle develops:

> EATING/DRINKING ➜ LOW BLOOD SUGAR ➜ MORE
> EATING/DRINKING ➜ AND SO IT GOES

And that soda probably has caffeine in it. Caffeine intensifies the body's response to epinephrine. Our young lady pretty quickly becomes a virtual invalid hooked on frequent sugar consumption to stave off crippling spells. It's far worse if she gets a blood-glucose monitor meant for diabetics, and starts tracking her up and down blood sugars and overeating carbohydrates as a result—triggering more spells!

Please, please, please, I beg you: if you aren't diabetic and haven't had gastric surgery and don't have an insulin-secreting tumor, I beg you, do not monitor your finger-stick blood sugars. The information only causes trouble. I promise. Nothing but anxiety and trouble. Everybody's blood sugar bounces up and down and sometimes gets low. That's normal. Your problem isn't that; your problem is your reaction to it. And your lousy diet of course.

I mention all this here because the excessive carbohydrate feeding, resulting from reactive hypoglycemia, will eventually cause weight gain. In my experience, this scenario occurs in two kinds of patients: (1) thin young women with anxious personalities (epinephrine primed to pour out), who also have very little muscle mass, meaning less glycogen is available to keep sugar levels up, and (2) obese, insulin-resistant patients on the verge of type 2 diabetes. The latter pump out a lot of insulin, still more or less effective, causing wide, uncomfortable swings in blood sugar.

The answer?

First—don't have a glucose tolerance test done—never, never, never helpful.

Second—switch to a low-glycemic-index diet.

Also—cut caffeine.

And truthfully just understanding what's happening blunts the fear and epinephrine release, and thus the symptoms. This is literally a disease that can be cured with a conversation.

If none of that works, stick with the low-GX diet but eat six small meals per day—lessening the glycemic load at any one time and providing a pretty steady source of calories to smooth out sugar fluctuations.

That's it.

I explain and recommend all of that and I literally never see these patients again.

I choose to think that means they got better...*right?*

21

IMBIBING: VICE, OR ELIXIR OF LIFE?

Where does alcohol fit in to weight management?

First, and most basically—beers, wines, and distilled spirits are a source of calories. A significant source. So, all other pros, cons, risks and benefits aside, alcohol-containing (specifically *ethanol*-containing) beverages need to be considered alongside all other food and caloric-liquid consumption, and limited accordingly, in view of your overall nutritional plan, and weight-regulating goals.

ETHANOL METABOLISM

Ethanol is converted first to *acetaldehyde*, then *acetate*, both steps energy liberating, that is, calorie producing. Acetate is converted to our old friend *acetyl-CoA*, which we called earlier the *central substance in human metabolism*, the crossroads of all the major metabolic pathways. It can enter the Krebs cycle to release more calories, or be converted to other substances, including triglycerides and cholesterol. Thus, in spite of its unique properties, on one level ethanol is no different, better or worse, and just as flexible, as many other bioenergetic nutrients. In fact, compared to other macronutrients, it's about average in terms of actual calorie content: a gram of ethanol yields seven calories, a gram of protein or carbohydrate, four, and one of fat, nine calories.

Calories by Type

That isn't the whole story, however, of energy intake attributable to alcoholic beverages. The various beers, wines, and spirits all contain differing amounts of sugar, as well as ethanol, and every gram of sugar adds four calories to the seven per gram derived from the alcohol. For medical purposes, a *standard drink* is defined as a serving containing 14 grams of ethanol: thus, one drink of beer is 12 ounces, one of wine, approximately 4 ounces, and distilled spirits (gin, rum, vodka, whiskey), one *jigger*, or 1.5 ounces. The number of grams of carbohydrates in a serving of these beverages varies, but averages around 13 for beer (3 to 8 for light beer), a range of 4 to 14 for wines (reds and other drier wines, less sugar, sweeter dessert wines, sherries, and so forth, more sugar), and a trace amount for spirits. Cocktails add all manner of sweet mixers for the purpose of masking the strong flavors of straight liquors, and may have considerable carbohydrate content, up to 9 grams according to one medical text (varying widely, of course), with a total calorie count possibly exceeding two hundred—more than a can of Mountain Dew. There's even fat in some cocktails, a Brandy Alexander, for instance, which includes heavy cream and a sweet chocolate liqueur.

So, depending on variety, how it's prepared, what quantities, alcoholic beverages may be either a relatively high-, or a relatively low-calorie segment of one's diet. My own take is that, with respect to obesity and diabetes, "adult beverages," consumed in moderation, are no worse than, and often healthier than the sugary sodas, sweet teas, and syrup-and-sugar-and-cream-laden vente-sized coffee drinks so ubiquitous today. An obvious exception would be heavily sweetened cocktails, which I advise avoiding to the same degree I advise avoiding any sugary drink, especially in frequent or sizeable servings.

From least unhealthy to most unhealthy—focusing on weight issues, not on intoxicating effects—I rank order alcoholic beverages as follows: (1) in moderation, straight or water-diluted distilled spirits (e.g., Scotch and water, bourbon on the rocks); (2) traditional dry cocktails—again, in moderation—such as the classic martini (I emphasize *dry*, meaning little vermouth, limiting sugar intake, and *traditional*, meaning no cranberry juice or apples or the like); (3) red or white wine; (5) beer.

The Special Case of Light Beer

I omitted from the ranking above *light beers*, which have about the same calorie content per serving as straight distilled liquors; that is, tied for best in our ranking based on calories.

However, light beers violate my quality-not-quantity rule.

They have roughly the same alcohol content as regular beer, but something like a fourth the carbohydrates. They are just as intoxicating, with fewer calories, throwing them in the same somewhat-disreputable, best-bypassed category, to my thinking, as diet soda. Remember those Miller Lite "Great Taste...Less Filling!" television commercials? (called the eighth-best advertising campaign in history.) Funny ads—my father liked the one with Mickey Spillane—but two problems:

What are they putting in to make it *taste great* despite a fourth the carbs? (In 1982, the Center for Science in the Public Interest reported propylene glycol, corn syrup, and seaweed extract, among other ingredients not normally found in beer.) And, if they are less filling, the average Joe and Josephine will drink more bottles of them in a sitting than regular beers, which is of course what the manufacturers and ad agencies want. Unfortunately, Joe and Josephine are drinking more alcohol, and probably more calories when they drink more of that "less filling" light beer.

Let's be conservative and say the guy who would have drunk one regular beer, instead drinks two light beers. Either because he thinks he's drinking something healthier, or because he's simply less satisfied by one bottle of the light product. That takes him from 13 grams ethanol, 13 grams carbohydrate, and 148 calories, to 24 grams ethanol, 6 grams carbs, and 192 calories. His "healthier" alternative gave him 84 percent more ethanol, less than half the sugar, but 30 percent more calories overall—meaning his blood sugar might be lower, if he has diabetes, but he's drunker and perhaps more likely to gain weight.

I, personally, feel very full and satisfied after one bottle of a hoppy premium pilsner from Germany, and you couldn't drag me to the refrigerator to get another. As it should be.

Light beer is another entity unleashed by the food-and-beverage industry on the unsuspecting American public (not *innocent*, but definitely *unsuspecting*), ostensibly "better" for us, but which ends up making us less satisfied and more prone to overconsumption—a plague on society, best avoided. If you're going to drink beer, drink good beer, or at least real beer.

And both your appetite and wallet will probably guide you to drink less.

BEYOND CALORIE COUNTING

We all know there are downsides to ethanol consumption beyond calories. Alcohol contributes to 79,000 deaths and $223.5 billion in societal costs annually in the United States, according to Peter D. Friedmann, MD, of Brown University medical school, in a 2013 *New England Journal of Medicine* paper: a counterpoint to the largely positive recent tone of the medical literature on moderate ethanol use. It is good to be reminded that less-responsible, less-restrained ethanol use is unquestionably a destroyer of lives.

The intoxicating effects of ethanol on the brain are universally known, and in moderation can be pleasant, even beneficial. Beyond a blood alcohol of, say, 0.04 percent, however, a continuum of negative effects on neuromuscular function ensue that increase in proportion to alcohol levels, starting with exaggerated emotions and behaviors, and impaired alertness and judgment, progressing to dangerous impairment of the ability to operate a motor vehicle, then to nausea, vomiting, blackouts, eventually to coma, even death.

Chronic heavy ethanol consumption—defined as *more than 14 standard drinks per week for men under 65, and seven for women and men over age 65 (current guidelines also stipulate no more than four drinks in any given day for younger men, three for women and men over 65)*—is associated with numerous poor outcomes. These include: shortened life span, violent behavior, liver disease, brain damage including dementia and loss of coordination, cardiovascular disease (coronary disease, stroke, congestive heart failure, atrial fibrillation), various endocrine disorders, including impaired sexual function and fertility, and thinning of the bones, and various cancers, including those of the esophagus, throat, liver, pancreas, prostate, colon, and breast. Unlike what has been observed for cardiovascular disease, no degree of ethanol consumption seems beneficial for cancer prevention.

Breast cancer is one of our greatest concerns. A recent cover story in *ACP Internist* cited Dr. Arthur Klatsky of Kaiser Permanente Northern California, saying, "The increased risk of breast cancer in moderate female drinkers outweighs any of the cardiovascular benefit of alcohol in women younger than age 50, but in postmenopausal women the cardiovascular benefit for total mortality outweighs the breast cancer risk."

Thus, it would be a mistake to dismiss the potential negative impacts of ethanol use on the individual and society. In moderation, however, there are benefits, and to dismiss them, too, would be a mistake. Ethanol is no different from any pharmaceutical with or without a prescription, in that to a point there are positive effects, but overdoses can have negative, even fatal consequences.

There are reasons, by the way, beyond simply body mass, for the guidelines defining safe ethanol consumption in women as roughly half that of men. Women have less body water than men owing to higher body-fat percentages (fat displaces water); therefore there is less volume to dilute the ethanol in. Women also have lower levels of the enzyme that metabolizes ethanol. Thus, given the same amount consumed per pound of body weight, a woman will experience a higher blood alcohol concentration than a man.

Who Should Avoid Ethanol?

I would not encourage anybody with a personal history of alcohol addiction, and possibly other substance-abuse disorders to use ethanol. A strong family history of abuse also warrants caution. Certainly ethanol should be avoided when there is significant chronic liver disease—alcohol related or not—or significant dementia, and in pregnancy. Severe osteoporosis (thin bones) can worsen with moderate to heavy ethanol use. Other conditions in which abstinence is advised are poorly controlled hypertension, peptic ulcer disease, many types of cancer, and some mental-health disorders such as anxiety or depression. Persons with a strong family history of cancer, or otherwise at high risk of cancer are advised to abstain. Obviously the intoxicating effects of ethanol on judgment and reaction time should be taken into account by those operating heavy machinery, and driving or piloting vehicles for a living. *Ethanol is implicated in one-third of all fatal traffic accidents.*

Is There an Upside?

Those precautions aside, ethanol consumption has benefits, and according to Dr. Walter Willett of the Harvard School of Public Health, "is probably good for most people."

Mortality rates plotted against ethanol use show a J-shaped curve: that is, starting out high, dipping, then rising again. In other words, both low and high ethanol intakes are associated with higher death rates, while users in the middle live longer. Provided the servings-per-week recommendations are not exceeded, it is well established that moderate ethanol consumption, compared to abstinence, protects against heart attacks, sudden cardiac death (in women taking one-half to one drink per day, 36 percent lower rate than abstainers), and the most common type of stroke, by raising HDL ("good") cholesterol, lowering the worst subtype of LDL ("bad") cholesterol, and reducing clot formation. Ethanol releases *adiponectin*, a fat-cell hormone, that reduces insulin resistance and inflammation, and protects against cardiovascular disease. Accordingly, reasonable ethanol consumption is associated with up to a 30 percent reduction in diabetes rates, compared with no, or higher levels of drinking. Other studies have suggested protection against Alzheimer's disease, rheumatoid arthritis, even the common cold. (My father, who drank more than was good for him, often boasted: "Do you know how long it's been since I had a cold?")

Diabetes + Alcohol = ?

We have noted that moderate ethanol intake improves insulin sensitivity (that is, lowers insulin resistance) and protects against type 2 diabetes. I believe that—as I similarly proposed with coffee— alcoholic beverages can be a healthier, less obesogenic, less diabetogenic alternative to sugary sodas, perhaps even diet sodas. But while coffee drunk black is always calorie free, alcoholic drinks always contain some calories owing to ethanol, and often more from carbohydrates.

Thus, alcoholic beverages are only beneficial for obesity prevention and management (part, not the whole, of the diabetes benefit) if consumed in a way that avoids excessive calories. Just as syrup-and-cream-laden coffee probably negates any benefit of the coffee, so might a sugar-heavy cocktail—a Long Island Iced Tea (270 calories, 32 carb grams), for example, or Cosmopolitan (215 calories, 12 carb grams), for example—negate any ethanol benefit.

For the record: The American Diabetes Association's 2013 guidelines state:

> If adults with diabetes choose to use alcohol, they should limit intake to a moderate amount (one drink per day or less for adult women and two drinks per day or less for adult men).

This is largely consistent with the guidelines for all younger, non-diabetic healthy adults. In other words, overall, ethanol is not worse for diabetics than for the general population. In fact a number of studies document improved blood-sugar control with moderate alcohol consumption.

That said, ethanol metabolism does interfere with *gluconeogenesis*, the process whereby glucose is released into the bloodstream from the liver, for prevention of and recovery from hypoglycemia. Therefore, heavy ethanol use, not recommended for anyone, can help trigger life-threatening hypoglycemia in diabetics at risk of it by virtue of taking insulin or certain pills that might cause blood sugar to drop excessively. Fortunately, as stated earlier, many newer drugs for diabetes don't carry hypoglycemia as a risk.

For diabetics on insulin or pills that can cause hypoglycemia, however, the combination of heavy drinking and not eating—a behavior pattern in some serious alcoholics—can be deadly.

Like many aspects of medicine, the effect of ethanol on gluconeogenesis has both risks and benefits that require balance. We've said that interference with gluconeogenesis can lead to dangerous low blood sugars. We also have said that average glycemic control is better (that is, blood sugars are lower) in diabetic ethanol users. And part of the explanation for that is the interference with gluconeogenesis. For you see, this liver glucose release often goes haywire in type 2 diabetes and is a big part of what drives high blood sugars and poor control. So, a little bit of gluconeogenesis interference is good, while a lot can be bad.

Wine Premium?

Much has been made of the supposed advantages of red wine over other alcoholic beverages, owing to its containing resveratrol and other antioxidants that help prevent heart disease. Current clinical guidelines, however, *make no distinction between red and white wine and other types of alcoholic beverages*. It's the ethanol content that matters, not the form. Any benefit from resveratrol is probably overstated, and would require higher than practical levels of intake.

CONCLUSION

If you do drink alcoholic beverages, don't beat yourself up about it being the bad habit of its reputation—just keep the intake light to moderate. If you don't, especially if you have religious or legitimate medical reasons for abstaining, then don't start. A quality exercise program is probably as good.

On the other hand, if you are only abstaining because you believe the myth that ethanol is nothing but unhealthy, and if you have a high risk of cardiovascular disease, especially if your HDL cholesterol is low, then you might consider a daily drink or two. If you're a woman, the breast-cancer concern needs to be weighed, especially if your mother or sister have had breast cancer. It has been suggested that folate supplementation might protect against ethanol-enhanced breast cancer risk, and several studies support this, though there is not universal agreement. You should talk to your own doctor before going down that road—just remember there are risks and benefits to many things in life, including driving a car, flying, having a baby, and so on, and so on.

22

NOTHING (MUCH) TO BRAG ABOUT

This chapter is autobiographical, an illustration of how I have employed some of this book's principles in my own life, and the results. It is simply an illustration, which you might learn from, perhaps be inspired by. By inspiration, I don't mean to imply anything heroic. I recently heard a story of a middle-aged woman who changed her lifestyle after being diagnosed with breast cancer, and now, in her eighties, she's not only alive, but a competitive triathlete. I've accomplished nothing close to that impressive, but that's a good thing. It means if you find something in my story you want to emulate, it ought to be relatively easy to meet or surpass my example. Also, while my health challenges, including weight issues, are relevant to topics covered in this book, they have been—I am happy to say—very much on the mild end of the spectrum. If you're reading this seeking help for obesity or diabetes, there is a good chance the outcomes I report from my situation are modest in comparison to what you will need to accomplish. In fact, the best lesson to take away from my story, I think, is nothing about a massive loss of poundage, but rather, that numerous and varied lifestyle changes are possible, and can be made to persist. For that reason I'm going to be fairly detailed, and honest, perhaps embarrassingly so, about my dietary habits.

My key habit—the foundation of my program, if there is a program here—is to stop and think about everything. Not take anything for granted, especially long-held assumptions, like supper always has to be the biggest meal, or bread is a staple food that always must be in the house, or accepted by the basketful at every restaurant meal.

Most of you, I imagine, are like me. I grew up with and lived most of my adult life with bread on every grocery list—mostly soft white bread, sometimes crusty loaves of French bread, or the like, instead of, or in addition to the soft bread. It's something you have to have, right? Not anymore, not in my house. A long-held, pretty-much society-wide assumption dashed. But wait—a patient said this to me the other day—"it's hard to make sandwiches without bread." Agreed.

But, do we need sandwiches? Not in my house. That's another of those long-held, pretty-much society-wide assumptions, that sandwiches, of whatever kind, fill an essential dietary niche. They don't. No one ever died for lack of two pieces of bread to encase some other hardy food. That's what I mean by stopping and thinking, and questioning everything.

That takes time and focus; it means being ready for and committed to change. Not everyone is ready, all the time. It probably means setting aside, or waiting until you can set aside, other overwhelming concerns and distractions. If you are going through a divorce, or serious financial crisis, now may not be the time. But if you are committed to improving your health, especially if you already are obese or have diabetes, there will need to come a point when making big lifestyle changes does take priority over or at least right alongside other important aspects of life, like work, and children. The alternative is a gradual deterioration of your health, the development of complications of obesity and/or diabetes, to the point that no therapy (lifestyle, drug, or surgery) will ever bring you fully back.

For when you are ready, here's my example—submitted, to quote the Rod Sterling, for your approval…

MY STORY

I am, as of this writing, 52 years old. I have a strong family history of type 2 diabetes, including my father, his sister, their mother, and my paternal second cousin. I've never smoked. I've been generally healthy and moderately active, throughout my life, though never what anyone would label athletic. Prior to my early thirties, I intermittently pursued running, bicycling, and weightlifting, at low intensities and durations, often limited by shortness of breath and fatigue. I've never been overweight or obese by any objective standard. The most I recall weighing is 148 pounds, giving me a personal-high BMI of just under 25.

I think it remarkable, frankly, that my BMI never exceeded that generally recognized upper limit of normal, considering my diet over the years. I grew up in the "stroke-belt" of the South, the meals my mother cooked us being textbook examples of why the region was called that. As a child I drank several sugary sodas per day, mostly Mountain Dew (for whatever reason, "Dew" seems to be the preferred soft drink of my generation of physicians, and it ain't for its health benefits). It may be relevant to my tale that all this—my childhood and adolescence, that is—came before high-fructose corn syrup and the whole raft of modern no-calorie sodas, like Diet Mountain Dew, were invented.

I ate a lot of fried food, and fast-food hamburgers. In fact, until recent years I was a fairly heavy consumer of fast food, though never a "supersizer." As a medical resident, nights on call, my typical supper was a small pan pizza with extra cheese (*small*, not *personal*—that's a lot of pizza for one person!). I have always eaten too-little fruit. Salads, yes, but covered with cheese, bacon, fat-laden dressings. Red meat? Yep. On the plus side, I was never a big candy, cookie, or Twinkie-type snacker—that life-long Krispy-Kreme habit aside. In first grade, I sneaked the Twinkies my mother put in my *Lost in Space* lunchbox in the trash. I was a rather late and gradual adopter of alcoholic beverages: close to age thirty before I began to consume beer with any regularity, late thirties for wine, later still anything stronger.

In short, for much of my life, my diet, a few saving graces aside, was basically deplorable. Similarly, for the first two-thirds of my life, my physical activity, while never fully sedentary, was no great shakes either.

Yet my BMI has never yet exceeded 25.

Partly for this reason, I became an early and enthusiastic believer—in stark opposition at the time to mainstream endocrinology opinion—in low-glycemic-index/low-carbohydrate diets. I have long observed that, while I have been a fairly heavy consumer of fat and red meat, I have tended to limit carbohydrates, especially foods marketed as "fat free." Don't misunderstand: no bragging here about my habits over the years. I am merely reporting, and feeling lucky that I don't have more serious medical problems today than I do.

And because I don't—and granted I am only an experiment of one, not the stuff of scientific dogma—I believe in the glycemic index, at least for those with (like me) a family history of diabetes, and I believe there to be pervasive societal and food-industry issues, impacting the obesity and diabetes epidemics, which did not exist when I was a child and young adult. I did watch too much TV growing up, but I also played outside, and played inside with toys that spurred my imagination. I read more than average, even for the time. No computers, video games, mobile technology (decades before their time). I was not exposed to high-fructose corn syrup, nor diet drinks, from an early age, as children today often are.

Turning Points

I identify three watershed events in my, if you will, *personal metabolic journey.*

The first came about age 30. I was diagnosed with hypothyroidism and began taking daily Synthroid (thyroid hormone) and have remained on it since. I credit that with eliminating the mild chronic fatigue that had long limited my exercise.

Second, about age 34, I was divorced, and a female coworker and friend (who later set me up with Susan, my current wife of, now, fifteen years) encouraged me in a more aggressive physical-fitness program. Despite some effort, even on thyroid pills, I had never managed to push my endurance beyond running more than, say, three-quarters of a mile. To get over that hump I went to a gym before work, using a stair-climber for thirty minutes, gradually increasing exertion levels. This improved my conditioning and eventually I transitioned to running three miles in thirty minutes, three times per week. I largely continued this habit for the next ten years. I no longer run but walk a lot, briskly, ride an exercise bike, and lift weights regularly.

My third turning point came as I approached age 50, and was diagnosed simultaneously with hyperlipidemia and type 2 diabetes.

(Just as my BMI challenges have been mild, my diabetes has never been severe either, nor even requiring of medication. That said, it has always manifested with high fasting blood sugars alone, no high after-meal levels. That might sound good, and it is to a point. However, fasting hyperglycemia alone indicates a more dangerous metabolic profile. High post-meal sugars imply insulin *deficiency*; high fasting sugars imply insulin *resistance*, a derangement associated, as we know, with heart disease, stroke, and premature death. Thus, while my diabetes is by all measures mild, I am well motivated to control it.)

At the time I was diagnosed with diabetes and hyperlipidemia—the latter, for which, I take low-dose simvastatin with excellent results—my nutritional habits, which weren't pretty, included:

- No fruit
- Two hot dogs or a hamburger 2-3 times per week
- Fast food 1-2 times per week
- Mexican restaurant visits 1-2 times per week
- Bread, bread, bread.
- Half PBJ sandwiches as frequent snacks
- One big bag of potato chips per month (you read that right, even then, before I improved things—one per month)
- Occasional frozen waffles
- A full-sized frozen pizza with added cheese once weekly
- Pasta once weekly
- A big supper most evenings
- Beer and wine most days
- Several coffees a day, real sugar in the first, saccharin in the rest.
- One real and one diet Mountain Dew per day

At the time my hypothyroidism was diagnosed, in the early 1990s, I was at my lifetime high weight of 148 pounds. By the time diabetes and hyperlipidemia were diagnosed, twenty-odd years later, thyroid pills and regular exercise had brought me to a steady 140 to 142 pounds (a respectable 5 percent loss). At that point my blood chemistries were as follows:

- Fasting glucose   134 (>125 = diabetes)
- Hemoglobin A1C   5.8 (<7.0 = good diabetes control)
- Cholesterol   223
- HDL "good" cholesterol   49
- LDL "bad" cholesterol   158 (<100 is the goal)
- Non-HDL cholesterol   174 (<130 is good)
- Triglycerides   116
- Chol/HDL ratio   4.55 (lower is better and >4.5 ain't good)

I started simvastatin. My exercise continued, admittedly suboptimal, though fairly regular, and emphasizing, if anything, resistance training, weightlifting. I still don't lay claim to a perfect diet. It is, however, a fairly obsessive-compulsive diet, as was the bad one above. Meaning I stick pretty close to established habits and patterns. Physicians tend toward obsessive-compulsive personalities. Not everyone is wired that way, but it helps to cultivate a little compulsive behavior when trying to control weight and diabetes. Complete free-spirits (*undisciplined* would be a synonym for *free-*

spirited) may find more difficulty cutting calories and losing weight. Because, remember, in weight management, whatever works, whether it be diet, exercise, or pills, must be continued long term. Obsessive-compulsiveness fosters that.

Anyway—ideal or not—I made big changes.

And if I can, you can:

- I went from no fruit to several servings of fresh, not canned, fruit per week.
- No hot dogs and hamburgers at home—having them means a trip to a restaurant, which I might do for that purpose 1-2 times per month.
- No fast-food at work, I've stockpiled Lean Cuisines.
- I stopped the regular Mexican restaurant trips
- No bread in our house, which means no half PBJ's
- No potato chips or the like in our house
- No frozen waffles and if I want pancakes, I go out.
- No frozen pizzas
- Pasta maybe once a month
- No big supper except for special occasions, small snacks instead (deli meat, pickles, cheese), or soup or salad.
- Very rare beer
- Infrequent wine
- Two or three distilled-spirit drinks per day
- Other beverages:
  o One real Mountain Dew per day
  o Much black coffee without any sugar or other sweetener
  o Water
  o No diet soda ever—if I cheat, it's with a real soft drink, nothing diet—I'm a strong believer in that.
- Breakfast:
  o At work:
    ▪ One breakfast bar, or:
    ▪ More recently, one of those Lean Cuisines I have stockpiled (thinking "outside the box," no pun intended, because these are not traditional breakfast entrées)
  o At home:
    ▪ Bran cereal with skim milk, or:
    ▪ Two eggs sunny-side up cooked in olive oil, with fresh fruit.
- Lunch is my main meal:
  o At work:
    ▪ Lean Cuisine, or:
    ▪ A careful selection from whatever the pharmaceutical salesperson brings to the office (this is my biggest challenge, placing choices I might automatically exclude in too-easy reach—my willpower is not ironclad.)
  o At home:
    ▪ Homemade tuna or egg salad, alone or atop lettuce (remember,

no bread in the house), or:

- Soup, or:
- A green salad, no croutons, generally some bottled vinaigrette in modest amounts, though I don't rule out any dressing, so long as HFCS isn't an ingredient.
  - o Occasional lunches out vary, but typically involve sushi or Thai, or some other Asian cuisine, which I mention because, despite being a committed carnivore, I often choose vegetables only for stir-fry dishes rather than those bits of probably low-quality chicken, pork, or beef; this might be part of a "vegetarian day."
- Lastly, I do eat meat, including red meat, but less of it than once I did (in fact, like hamburgers and hot dogs, we don't generally have steaks at home; my top guilty pleasure is a late afternoon steakhouse dinner, perhaps a couple of times per month, half the steak going home for the next day's lunch [and the blonde dog Emma on the porch gets the bone!]).

The Results

I've made big changes, cutting out much unhealthy consumption. Many would consider what I'm still doing unhealthy, and I'm not suggesting you copy me, but I hope this example proves big changes are possible. Einstein's oft-quoted definition of *insanity* was: doing the same thing over and over, expecting a different result. Even if you quibble with my diet, I hold it up as an example of three very positive changes: (1) portion size, (2) frequency, and (3) quality.

I'm eating less of everything. Higher-calorie, higher-fat foods (like beefsteak, fried chicken) are occasional treats, not daily staples (Thomas Jefferson said meat should be a seasoning, not a course). And I eat more natural, less processed, less artificial foods.

What's been the result of those changes, plus low-dose simvastatin?

Today I weigh 125 pounds (12 percent down from the point the diet started, almost 16 percent from my peak adult weight). I've never felt better. I've lost four inches from my waist. Let's look at that blood work again, compared to the first set, 27 months earlier (old numbers on the left):

- Fasting glucose — 134 — 134
- Hemoglobin A1C — 5.8 — 5.7
- Cholesterol — 223 — 155
- HDL "good" cholesterol — 49 — 67
- LDL "bad" cholesterol — 158 — 82
- Non-HDL cholesterol — 174 — 88
- Triglycerides — 116 — 53

- Chol/HDL ratio   4.55   2.31

My diabetes didn't improve much, but nor did it worsen, which type 2 diabetes is wont to do, and I'm still on no medication for that condition. And, I think it intriguing, and illustrative, that if I'm avoiding anything, it's carbohydrates in general, sugar in particular, and if I am nutritionally liberal about anything it is fat. Yet, my Chol/HDL ratio (an estimate of heart-attack and stroke risk) is almost exactly half where it started, as is my LDL, and non-HDL cholesterol, which is a sort of global estimate of harmful lipoprotein fractions.

Much of the lipid benefit did come from the simvastatin, data which I've not shown, for brevity. Nevertheless, even after the initial impact of the drug, there came a further 20 percent improvement in the Chol/HDL ratio (2.88 to 2.31) owing only to lifestyle change and weight loss. In fact, the drug hardly budged my HDL from its baseline of 49 (it went to 50), yet lifestyle changes, mainly I suspect, shifting from beer and wine, toward distilled spirits, raised my HDL to 67, a number I rarely see in men (higher HDLs are better).

It is now about a year since that second set of numbers and I have just obtained another battery of tests. I have made no substantial changes in lifestyle habits or medications in the intervening year, but have maintained fairly faithfully the efforts outlined. Thus, any further changes reflect duration of effort, rather than difference in quality or quantity of effort. In other words, the benefits of perseverance, the eating of the elephant a bite at a time.

My weight, incidentally, has not changed, still averaging 125.

My fasting blood glucose is now 117, down from 134.

The hemoglobin A1c (average blood sugar) has continued its gradual decline, now 5.6.

I won't give all the cholesterol numbers, but the Chol/HDL ratio further improved to 2.26, the HDL to a whopping 72, the LDL to 80.

OPTIMISM FOR THE FUTURE?

In an updated edition perhaps I can report more improvements, because at long last I'm cutting back even more on sugary beverages. I was down to, as I reported, one daily 12-ounce, HFCS-sweetened Mountain Dew. Now, once a week or so, I abstain, substituting V8 juice (ounce for ounce, 60% fewer calories, 80% less sugar, it's got fiber, but—it's also got 14 times more sodium, so it's not an everyday solution to a "Dew" habit). Also, about half the time I substitute a 7.5-oz. can of soda, which I'm finding to be readily available of late, even at Walmart, to industry's credit. As we've discussed, I don't believe they are marketing such products primarily out of concern for public health. They are doing it because they know we are concerned about public health, and they want our business, and that's fine. Perhaps this is reason for optimism, reassurance that change is possible if we want it and demand it, and purchase it, rather than just going along with what we are accustomed to and what is thrust in front of us. Walmart could if it wanted, be a bastion of unhealthy, highly processed foods. Instead I've observed a trend toward better quality products on its shelves, more organic foods even. This is because the mainstream public, their customer base, is demanding it and supporting it.

There is some role for legislative action in the regulation of mass food-and-beverage marketing and retailing, but my hope is that most of what must be accomplished in the battle against diabetes and obesity can be through personal choice, and personal education, and the consumer-driven, free-enterprise system. Remember, price goes down where demand goes up.

23

STRATEGIC THINKING

This concluding chapter will summarize my approach to achieving and maintaining a healthy body weight—which above all, recognizes and addresses a broad variability in the causes of obesity from one individual to another, and in their responses to various therapies. In short, what works for one person is unlikely to work as well, if at all, in another.

I am using the term *strategy* rather than *plan*.

A plan is "a method for achieving an end," or "a detailed formulation of a program of action." Implying something pretty limited and specific. There is no weight-loss plan here like so many books and gurus purport to provide. There is no such thing—not one anyway, that works for all or most people. A *strategy*, as I use the term, is: "the art of devising or employing plans toward a goal." Thus, a strategy involves multiple plans, and different groups of plans for different cases. How do we know which plans go with which case? We don't. We sometimes can make educated guesses, like a low-glycemic-index diet might work better when there is a family history of type 2 diabetes, but not always. The best plan is the one that works. Meaning trial and error. Being flexible. Thinking outside the box.

Quoting a recent *New England Journal of Medicine*: "Diets...very effectively reduce weight, but trying to go on a diet or recommending that someone go on a diet generally does not work well in the long-term...This seemingly obvious distinction is often missed..."

In other words, the physics of weight loss is simple. Intake fewer calories than you burn off and you will lose weight. The rub being, that's harder to do in real life than most of us realize. Tipping the metabolic teeter-tooter the right way, keeping it tipped, then later keeping it level, is easier said than done. The *physics* is simple; the *physiology* is not. The physiology of obesity is complex and regulated, and much of it, including a big and variable chunk of daily energy expenditure, is not under the control of conscious human will.

If physiology runs roughshod over physics, then why do I bother detailing the physics? Because the physics is true and of practical relevance in one key respect:

If you gained it, you ate it or drank it.

Matter, body weight, is neither created nor destroyed. If your friend eats Food A, in quantity Y, and does not gain weight—great!—the complex and regulated physiology worked in her favor. If you then follow your friend and eat the same food in the same quantity, one of three things can happen, regardless of your friend's outcome: your weight might not change, or you might gain weight or lose weight. Whatever happens it will be largely the result of behind-the-scenes modulation of resting metabolic rate, largely in skeletal muscle, but also in brown adipose tissue. If your weight remained stable your body chose to burn those calories from Food A, or else some equal number of stored calories from some previous meal. If you lost weight, your body chose to burn some greater number of calories than what you ate of Food A, some or all of which came from some meal other that the Food A meal. If you gained weight, on the other hand, your body chose to store the calories from Food A, and/or failed to burn calories stored from previous meals.

There was not a single calorie—burned or stored—in that above discussion that was not eaten by you as a part of either the present Food A meal, or some prior meal. Your body can store or burn any calorie it wants, almost at a whim—it's not really a whim, but it might as well be for all we can control it. But it can't burn or store a calorie you didn't eat. I emphasize this, perhaps overly, for some of you, because as I alluded to in Chapter 1, a day doesn't go by I don't have a patient telling me she's gaining weight without "eating a thing," or some equivalent obvious untruism. No weight is ever gained that is not first swallowed—even if it is simply salt and water retention. To be misled into not accepting that fact irreparably damages the effort that must go into basic lifestyles changes—eating less, exercising more—that are the first step to any successful weight-management campaign.

Those basic simple lifestyle changes—"diet and exercise"—are the first step, the nidus, if you will, in my healthy-weight strategy. And if simple changes fail, that doesn't mean something is wrong, or that you can't eventually succeed. If I can bring any helpful, reassuring personal perspective from my own practice into this discussion, it is this: as an endocrinologist I see a broader spectrum of patients than many doctors. I see young otherwise healthy adults with mild thyroid problems, and I see elderly diabetics with multiple complex medical problems. Obviously I see patients with seemingly healthy BMIs, and I see many morbidly obese, with BMIs over forty or fifty. But there is not a segment of my patient population—regardless of age or BMI—from which I do not hear frustration about weight. Concern about gaining, inability to lose, how little has been lost relative to effort put in. I offer this perspective not to be critical, or ridiculing, but as a demonstration that you are not alone or unique if you have these feelings.

If simple diet and exercise changes fail, alter something—increase intensity, or try a different mix—or add other types of changes. All obesity treatments that work must ultimately lower the set point around which the brain slaves to maintain one's weight—otherwise you'll lose and gain it right back. Different things probably do that and they probably vary with the individual. My guess is that it typically takes something drastic: not just a shift from junk food to less junk food, but rather junk food to whole foods, for example. Drastic might mean use of anorectic drugs, or even bariatric surgery.

My healthy-weight strategy—which is fairly nutrition-centric, but acknowledges non-nutritional factors, like activity, sleep, what prescription drugs you're taking—boils down to starting with simple diet and exercise, making at least one drastic change, and after that add things and change things until you find something that works. Don't be afraid to use common sense, think for yourself, flout conventional wisdom. Don't get so bogged down in numbers, counting calories, that you miss the big picture. And don't get too grandiose or in too much of a hurry: small changes in BMI may be of more medical importance than large ones. Slow down your weight loss.

The tortoise beat the hare, after all.

The components of my strategy are further summarized as follows:

1. Eat less
2. Eat better

3. Eat smarter
4. Have a plan
5. Consider other factors

EAT LESS

Most Americans eat too much. If you weigh more than you want (assuming you don't have an eating disorder) and you aren't progressing toward your goal, then eat and drink fewer calories. I don't care how much you've already cut, nor how you compare to anybody else, you can probably cut more and still survive it. Make it a habit to question every serving. Is it too big? Automatically cut it in half; take one instead of two. If you really didn't get enough, go back for more, but by that point you should feel fuller than when you started. Maybe you won't want the extra or you'll want less of it. Eating slowly helps too. And if you've cut, and cut some more, what's the worst that's likely to happen? You'll lose more weight than you intended and you'll have the pleasure of liberalizing your diet. Win:win!

EAT BETTER

Pay more for higher quality food, and more natural, less-processed whole foods, which are liable to be healthier, and more satisfying. And between enhanced satisfaction and higher cost, you'll automatically eat less. And if you do, in fact, eat less—to address the *What about the impoverished?* pushback—overall costs might not be that much higher, or not at all. Foods and beverages high in sugar should be avoided, which is especially, though not exclusively, true of high-fructose-corn-syrup-sweetened products.

EAT SMARTER

Healthy calorie consumption is complex. It requires thought, experimentation, trial and error, to create a nutritional lifestyle that works for your genetic metabolic profile and your preferences. If your personal preferences are obviously unhealthy—a daily big bag of potato chips, for instance—some modification is necessary. However, any long-term nutritional program that fails to incorporate to some degree your established habits, likes and dislikes, ethnic-food background, is doomed to failure. You should not go off following just any ol' fad diet. That's the simple thing to do. The easy way out, to read a book, follow it to the letter, and hope it works.

My bet is it won't, if some thought wasn't put into choosing or modifying the program based upon individual factors. Even if it does work, it won't last. I am, for example, a believer in low-glycemic-index diets, because I have diabetes and work with many diabetic patients. I think these plans (e.g., *Sugar Busters!*) work better for diabetics and those with a family history of type 2 diabetes than, say, a diet focused on fat. That's an example of selecting an approach based on one's genetic profile.

I advise taking with a grain of salt any and all simpleminded, universally accepted, not often questioned rules for what's healthy and what's not.

All fat is bad.

All sugar is bad.

Coffee's bad.

Alcohol is bad.

None of these statements is true. They might contain seeds of truth. A person with a history of serious alcoholism probably should avoid alcohol, not because alcohol is bad but because alcohol is bad for that individual. And just as people are diverse, so are these categories of food and beverages. Amount and type are important variables. A little sugar is fine for most and a lot is bad for most. A lot of trans fat is probably bad for most; a little olive oil in a salad dressing is probably good. Don't try to make something complicated into something simple.

Don't be led around by the nose by the food industry. Ignore their marketing tactics, ignore deals. Ignore healthy-eating hype on labels, like fat free or sugar free. *Natural*, let's be clear, is not, never has been, a synonym for *safe*. Skim the ingredients list of everything you buy.

HAVE A PLAN

Have an overall plan, and a daily plan. Weighing every day—getting either reinforcement or a red-flag about recent efforts—might help you formulate and follow that plan more effectively. Alan Lakein, an author of self-help books, said, "Failing to plan is planning to fail." Start out each day with a general idea of the what and where of each meal and major snack. It's like having a budget to get your finances in order. Get-out-of-debt guru Dave Ramsey says spend every dollar on paper before the month begins; I say eat and drink every calorie in your brain before the day begins. That doesn't mean you can't enjoy spontaneity, but it does mean when you do overindulge, an adjustment downward must be made either later that day or the next day. Very little should be a surprise, because when it is, it's not under control. I don't, for instance, think you should just eat when hungry. When you're hungry you eat more; you don't want to stack the deck against being able to limit overeating, and you don't want to let unexpected, unpredictable factors direct your eating. If you eat three meals or two meals or six meals—whatever—most every day, on time, regardless of hunger, then you will prevent hunger and impulse eating.

Two other issues should be in this plan:

Physical activity.

And sleep.

Most nights, get more than six hours, preferably seven to eight. Most weeks try to get two or three thirty-minute sessions of moderately intense endurance exercise, and on other days look for every opportunity to burn extra calories. And never ever look for ways to avoid burning calories. Remember: resistance training might be more important for your weight than endurance training. The more muscle you have, the more calories you'll burn, even at rest.

OTHER FACTORS

Don't take for granted your prescription medications. Many are weight promoting, including a number of diabetes drugs, beta-blockers, and antidepressants, and especially antipsychotics. Discuss these with your doctor(s). And think twice before taking any antibiotic; make sure it's really necessary and useful for what it's being prescribed for. Antibiotics don't treat viral upper respiratory infections, for instance, but they do alter the gut microbiota, promoting obesity. And for that matter, think just as hard about that next shot or course of steroids—they may be necessary, or they may not. We are an overmedicated society, and that is yet another contributor to the epidemic of obesity.

A WISE MAN

I first mentioned Michael Pollan, a premiere critic of the American diet and food industry, in Chapter 13. That was in the thick of our quality-not-quantity discussion—partly inspired by Pollan's writing—which got me accused of being an elitist by my mother-in-law after she edited a draft of this book. In subsequent drafts I've attempted to soften that message, but I couldn't purge it and be intellectually honest, or adequately address the topic of healthy eating. Understandably the notion of paying more for less raises hackles in some quarters, yet it is the lower-income segments of our society that tend to be most affected by obesity and obesity-related disease, partly due to their being forced to, or believing that they are forced to subsist on lower quality food-and-beverage products. I only mention all this because I got a chuckle reading a *Publishers Weekly* review of a new Michael Pollan book. The reviewer praised Pollan, but then added he was an *elitist!*

I will close with a list of principles abridged and paraphrased from Pollan's *New York Times Magazine* article "Unhappy Meals," published in January, 2007:

1. Eat nothing your great-great-grandmother wouldn't recognize as food
2. Avoid food products bearing health claims
3. Avoid food products containing unfamiliar, unpronounceable, overly numerous ingredients, or high-fructose corn syrup, all markers for highly processed foods.
4. Get out of the supermarket; no HFCS at the farmer's market, nor foods harvested long ago, far away.
5. Pay more, eat less.
6. Eat mostly plants.
7. Eat like the French, Japanese, Italians, Greeks. Any traditional food culture, and pay attention to *how* they eat: smaller portions, taking pleasure in eating. Fretting about food can't be healthy.
8. Cook. Plant a garden. Food shouldn't be cheap and easy.
9. Eat like an omnivore; diversity covers all nutritional bases.

Bon appetite!
And a martini toast to your good health!

APPENDIX A

THE PHYSICS OF OBESITY

Thanks to Albert Einstein, and the theory of relativity, we know mass and energy can be interconverted, each turned into the other, hence the term *mass-energy*, as used for example, in the *law of conservation of mass-energy*, discussed in Chapter 1. Mass is "congealed" energy; energy is "freed" mass.

For our purposes, discussing obesity and human energy balance, *mass* is equivalent to and interchangeable with *body weight*, and *energy* is equivalent to and interchangeable with *calories*. Therefore, since mass is energy in a different form, and vice versa, so too, body weight is calories in a different form, and calories are body weight in a different form. When we increase calorie intake, we increase weight; when we increase weight, we are storing increased calories that were taken in. Period, no way around that—provided we remember that body weight for obesity-management purposes involves all matter in our bodies other than water. Water is matter and has weight, but it has no calories. It does have energy in the physics sense—that "congealed-energy" business—but not in a biological sense. Our bodies never can tap into the energy locked up in water molecules.

The law of conservation of mass-energy—also known as the *first law of thermodynamics*, or what we have been calling, *the conservation law*—states the sum of energy plus mass in a closed system does not change. Mass and energy can change form (solid, liquid, gas, heat, light, and so on), but they can neither be created, nor destroyed. Now, the iconic equation "$E=mc^2$," defines the relationship between mass and energy. It says mass can disappear into energy, and defines how much energy one can get out of any substance of a given mass—quite a lot actually, that's how we get fission reactors and H-bombs. None of this violates the conservation law; matter is not destroyed in this process, and energy is not created. A certain amount of stuff is simply converted to a different form of the same stuff, and the total amount of stuff never changes.

In terms relevant to medicine and obesity, food is matter and it contains a certain amount of energy, which we call calories. Fat on our hips is also matter and can be converted to energy, which we call calories. When fatty acids, little energy-containing molecular packets, are released from fat tissue, and are metabolized by working muscle, the fat is not destroyed and the calories powering the work are not created; they are one and the same, just different forms of the same stuff. The mass in those free fatty acids is equal to the sum of the energy released plus the mass of whatever matter is left over—the molecular by-products of metabolism.

Now, I made a distinction in Chapter 1 between the *chemical energy* yielded during metabolism, and *nuclear*, or if you will, *relativistic* (i.e., related to the theory of relativity) *energy*. Chemical energy is the relatively small quantity of energy released when chemical bonds that link the atoms making up a molecule (a fatty-acid molecule, for example) are broken by enzymes in our cells. Nuclear energy is the much larger amount of energy released when individual atoms are split. No process in our bodies splits atoms, let's be clear on that. Everything we're dealing with in the medical/obesity arena is chemical energy.

The distinction I made in Chapter 1 to simplify the discussion, was to say that no mass is lost, destroyed, when nutrients are metabolized to chemical energy. I made that point to bolster the notion that nothing is created nor destroyed in human metabolism. No weight is gained that wasn't swallowed, nor is any weight lost that doesn't somehow physically leave the body—breathed out, urinated out, sweated out, defecated out.

That statement is true for any conceivable practical purpose of ours as a doctor and a patient. Body weight is neither created nor destroyed. At this point though I want to reintroduce the notion that matter does "disappear" whenever energy is "produced." Matter is "destroyed" when energy is "created." And energy is "destroyed" when matter is "created." The two are interchangeable. The total of the two never changes. That is what the law of conservation of mass-energy is really telling us.

But, the relationship between matter and energy is defined by the theory-of-relativity equation $E=mc^2$, where "E" is energy, "m" is mass, or matter, and "c" is the speed of light. Now, the speed of light is a huge number. And if you square a huge number, you get a phenomenally gigantic number, right? Meaning tiny masses of matter equal enormous amounts of energy and vice versa. This is how a single bomb dropped on Hiroshima in 1945 killed 70,000 people and destroyed 4.5 square miles of a modern city.

The point being, in this chemical-energy realm of human metabolism, when energy is released by breaking covalent bonds, mass is lost from the metabolites. It has to be; the energy can't come from nothing. It's just that the amount of mass lost is infinitesimally small, so small it can't be measured, not by anything practical like a bathroom scale. If it weren't incredibly small, then the amount of energy produced—which is more than the mass by a factor of the square of the speed of light—would cause us to burst into flames as we walk down the street, or something equally violent and grisly.

Logic and science dictate that the opposite must also be true. In order for mass to appear in the body—without it first being swallowed in the form of some solid or liquid, as some of my patients seem to truly believe can happen—it would have to be taken in as energy by some subliminal route, then converted to mass. Why would it have to be energy? The only significant access to the body's metabolic machinery for solids and liquids is the mouth. Agreed? The only other form that mass can take is gaseous. Gases do enter the body, via the respiratory tract, and do have a major role in metabolism. But as we discussed in Chapter 1, respiratory gas exchange, oxygen in/carbon dioxide out, is a weight losing proposition, any way you cut it. In fact, the only conceivable retention of weight-giving mass by the body from inhaled air is the small portion of oxygen that gets converted to water. Even if that is retained, it's water, not fat, and remember fat is all we care about from the standpoint of obesity and obesity-related disease. What about that 79 or so percent of the atmosphere that is nitrogen? Completely inert, atmospheric nitrogen cannot be metabolically incorporated into the human body (the process is called *fixation* and only bacteria can do it). Gaseous nitrogen is dissolved in the bloodstream, and would contribute a tiny amount to body weight, but the amount never changes as long as we remain relatively close to the surface of the earth. (This is an issue for scuba divers and astronauts, mainly, but even then, weight is never the concern.)

So, the only hypothetical way for mass to be gained by the body other than via the stomach would be for energy to be somehow taken in directly, in the form of energy. The problem is, for such a hypothetical process to occur, for it to increase one's body weight enough to measure it on a bathroom scale, the amount of energy taken in would have to be huge. Don't forget, we're talking about $E=mc^2$ here. Referring to our high-school algebra, the amount of mass gained by such a process would be determined by the formula $m=E/c^2$. In other words, the amount of mass produced would be the energy taken in *divided by* an enormous number (the speed of light squared). In order, therefore, to gain an amount of weight measureable on your scale, or mine in my office, the amount of energy that would have to somehow be absorbed into the body, as energy, would be huge. The process would cataclysmic—we wouldn't survive it. We'd be burned to a crisp or something. At the very least, you'd know it if it was happening.

Again, the point of all this is to say that nothing can increase the mass of the human body—increase body weight—other than mass that is swallowed. There is no other possible source. Yes, sunlight interacts with human skin to produce Vitamin D and increase melanin (skin pigment), but these are not processes involved with energy metabolism. In fact, more Vitamin D seems to, if anything, promote a healthy body weight, not obesity. Humans, nay all animals, are incapable of deriving usable energy from sunlight, as of course plants and certain bacteria do by way of *photosynthesis*.

Food eaten contains mass and energy, weight and calories. Once eaten, the total mass and energy in food gets split up, not destroyed, split up, so that if you could ever bring it all back together it would weigh the same as it started out on the plate. Let's say we're talking about exactly a half-pound total of a baked potato topped with butter, sour cream, bacon and chives, and this half-pound mix of digestible carbohydrate, fiber, fat, protein, and water gets eaten. Some of it will be eliminated from the body as stool and urine (Fate #1). Some of it will be retained by the body to build muscle, heal wounds, grow hair, to name a few structural possibilities (Fate #2). Some will be used as energy to power, mostly, muscles and the brain (Fate #3). And finally some will be stored in fat tissue, and a few other locations, to be later used as energy (Fate#4). If we could somehow recover all of this in pure form, make four little piles, labeled *Stuff That Went Through Fate#1*, *Stuff That Went Through Fate#2*, and so forth, and weighed each pile exactly, the sum of the weights of the four piles would equal exactly a half-pound.

Nothing created nor destroyed.

It's been changed. I imagine those four piles look utterly disgusting, compared to that delectable baked potato. But when all is said and done the human body neither created nor destroyed anything.

By the way, if we actually did this experiment and had the gear and know-how to measure the energy (in ergs) yielded out of Fate#3, we could in fact calculate using $E=mc^2$ the exact mass (in grams) of food that "vanished" in the yielding of that energy. That figure would constitute a small portion of the *Stuff That Went Through Fate#3* term in last paragraph's arithmetic problem, in which everything adds up to a half-pound. The complete Fate#3 term would be: *Energy Yielded (in ergs) plus By-Products of Energy Metabolism (in grams)*. The full equation would be: ½ pound baked potato = Fate#1 grams + Fate#2 grams + (Fate#3 ergs + Fate#3 grams) + Fate#4 grams = 1100 grams = ½ pound of a stinky mess.

Of course, we know we can ignore the ergs part of Fate#3 because in everyday experience the amount of matter changed into energy (or vice versa) is so small a fraction of the total mass of our bodies, that it cannot be detected. So, whether we measure Fate#3 ergs or not, you'll still end up with a half-pound, or something infinitesimally close. Thus, for practical medical purposes, when we say mass-energy is neither created nor destroyed, we can rephrase that statement into the simpler proposition: *body weight is neither created nor destroyed.*

Now there is another important piece of the conservation law we've ignored to this point.

"The sum of energy plus mass *in a closed system* does not change."

In a closed system—the entire process takes place within a sealed box, or entirely within the body of an organism. Are human beings closed systems?

Absolutely not.

We intake nutrients, water, and salts by mouth; sweat out water and salts; urinate out water and salts, some nutrients; we defecate, ejaculate, respire. Not a closed system. A very simple way of breaking down mass-energy handling by the body is as follows:

1. INGESTION—Food and beverages are swallowed
2. RETENTION—A portion of what is ingested is held onto
3. ELIMINATION—The rest is eliminated, mostly as stool and urine.

The first and third steps involve exchanges with the environment. These are open parts of the system. Step two is everything that happens to a meal or snack from the time it is ingested to the time it is eliminated. Step two takes place entirely within the human body, and therefore, is a closed system. What we are talking about here is the digestion and absorption of our meal, and its metabolism, such that it is either used directly for energy to do work or run some bodily function, or held onto in some more or less permanent way, serving as either the brick-and-mortar infrastructure of our bodies, or as energy storage, including fat. From the standpoint of obesity, it seems obvious the ingestion step is important. The retention step is also important. I would argue that the elimination step is not. There are medical problems involving constipation or fluid retention that might elevate weight, but these things are not obesity, which is, by definition, an excess of fat.

So, let's forget the elimination step.

That leaves *ingestion* and *retention* as key big-picture pieces in the pathophysiology of obesity. Ingestion is, obviously, more or less under voluntary control. It might not be totally so once complex appetite signals are thrown in, but to a point it is always a personal choice to eat or drink something or not. So, the ingestion piece is largely voluntary and open, a free exchange with the outside environment. The conservation law does not apply.

The retention piece is largely involuntary and closed. There are voluntary actions that might impact retention, the choice to exercise or not exercise, for example. But we can't decide directly how many calories are burned versus stored. Would that it were true.

What I'm saying is, between the points of ingestion and elimination, from mouth to anus, and to a lesser degree, to the urethra, the human body is a closed system and the conservation law does apply. Once a food is taken into the mouth, swallowed, it is impossible under the physical laws of the universe for the mass-energy of that food to increase. Once incorporated into the body, it is similarly impossible for the total weight of the structural features of the body—to include skeletal muscles and adipose tissue—to increase, except by the incorporation from the outside, of new ingested resources. For medically significant body weight to be gained, the closed part of the system must always engage the open part of the system.

The other physics principle relevant to obesity is *the second law of thermodynamics*, stating that there is a preferred direction for any process. The second law deals with *entropy*: the measure of a system's degree of disorder. As perfected by the German physicist Rudolf Clausius (1822–1888), the second law requires that all processes of change tend toward increasing entropy. Restated, the second law of thermodynamics asserts that *the entropy of the universe tends to maximum.*

This actually helps explain the paradox of obesity. Why it is seemingly so difficult, in spite of one's best efforts, to not gain weight. Put in the context of human weight control, weight gain is the anti-entropy. The more mass one can manage to pack into one's body, to be carried around and acted upon physiologically, the less entropy, more order, one has imposed upon one's little piece of the universe.* God's little acre, as it were.

The more entropy one has—that is, the greater the disorganization of one's body—the fewer energy resources might be readily available to be tapped in a crisis, the less efficiently the body might manage the processes of digestion, and toxin breakdown, and wound healing, to give a few examples. In other words, we can think of *weight gain as a state of decreasing entropy*, and *weight loss as a state of increasing entropy*. If we believe the second law, that entropy tends toward maximum, then any tendency for human beings to gain weight—which most, we well know, can do at the drop of a hat—is a tendency toward decreasing entropy.

Obesity thus flies in the face of the second law, which says entropy always wants to increase.

Are human beings above the second law of thermodynamics, a fundamental law of the universe? Of course not. Entropy, that tendency toward breakdown and disorder, does act inexorably on our bodies. Ask anyone dealing with aging, the progression toward feebleness and senility. We grow old and/or get sick, and we die. We get buried, everything scatters off in disorder. Entropy going through the roof, put bluntly. Our souls go off to Heaven, our flesh is consumed, carried off by all manner of microbe and vermin. Entropy wins, in the end. The second law does apply.

But for as long as we are alive and healthy, it is held at bay.

For life is, by definition, a low-entropy system: *a low entropy, potentially self-replicating, homeostatic system maintained by energy flow through*

---

* There is obviously a point of diminishing returns here: weight gain initially equates with good health (generally speaking, end-stage cancer patients don't gain weight, right?), and good health would imply low entropy. When weight gain, though, leads to obesity, and obesity-related diseases of increasing severity, then health declines and entropy increases.

it. Entropy wins in the long run, but just as Newton's physics stands corrected next to Einstein's, yet Newtonian laws work just fine in the narrow circumstances of our everyday lives, we, the physician and patient, wedged between birth and death, get to cheat. Human physiology—all living physiology—holds entropy off, for a while, but never forever. And that's a tough job for our bodies. Drastic measures are sometimes needed. Like, for example, planting an insatiable craving for Doritos in our minds, when really we'd prefer not to have anything right then.

It turns out that this powerful physiology of human energy balance is really rather blind. This complex and regulated system, with its incredible capacity to render moot, at least partially, at least temporarily, two fundamental laws of physics, doesn't know its own strength, doesn't know when to stop.

It is blind to the fact that it is living in an obesogenic vat we call the modern First World. It is a system hardwired to think the next Ethiopian famine is right around the corner, the next Japanese POW camp, the next Auschwitz, the next devastating malignant illness. None of which are impossible, but nor I pray, are they likely, for the foreseeable future, for the bulk of the patient population I serve.

Our bodies don't know that though.

They operate according to a genetically defined template that we are not yet able to reprogram. And until we can, obesity prevention and treatment will remain a worthy adversary.

APPENDIX B

KUHNIAN PHILOSOPHY, GLYCEMIC INDEX, & FLAWED RESEARCH?

It concerns me how the academic elite of medicine develop clinical-practice guidelines intended to direct the care given by other physicians, as well as to inform insurers what therapies and tests ought and ought not be covered. There is a special need for scrutiny in this era when legitimate cost-containment needs, coupled with the increasing influence of third party payers, like federal and state governments, and the massive private insurance industry—who prioritize costs often over the wants and needs of patients and their doctors—are driving "evidence-based medicine" and risk denying patients care and treatments not anointed by the "evidence."

By this I mean a certain treatment or test, unless called for by a few top docs, at major medical schools, in their published guidelines, or supported by excellently conducted research reported in a scientific journal, might not be available to real-world patients. Perhaps worse, I think young physicians come out of training cowed by these top experts, devaluing individual thoughts and practice styles, subjugating them to evidence-based ("cookbook") medicine. It pains me to feel the need to remind us all that every licensed medical doctor has an undergraduate degree, a four-year medical degree, and usually three-to-five-or-more years post-graduate training. I'm not saying that physician quality doesn't vary—no system is perfect—but all such professionals should be well trained enough to formulate their own preferred ways of managing patients within a range of acceptable options, if encouraged, allowed, and paid to do so, which they are often, these days, not.

Don't misunderstand me. Well-conducted research and peer-reviewed papers and clinical-practice guidelines are all necessary to good medicine. Good doctors learn every day of their practice, throughout their careers. And of course it goes without saying that scientific knowledge in all fields, medicine not least of all, is constantly, acceleratingly expanding. But once clinically relevant information is out there, it should be the independent physician who primarily sorts out how to apply that data to each unique patient, and episode of care. No matter how good the research and conclusions, all the variables confounding a real-world situation can never be fully anticipated. And even if evidence-based medicine's answers could be accepted as 100 percent valid—does it seem likely there could ever be adequate evidence available, published to answer every question faced by every physician every day?

The original question from the text leading me to this discussion was:

Why did it take until less than ten years ago for low-glycemic-index dieting to be taken scientifically seriously? I don't mean that it had to be accepted by all doctors and clinical dietitians—healthy skepticism is, after all, one of the traditions and underpinning of Hippocratic medicine. But this question of low-fat versus low-carb diets was not for many years viewed open-mindedly by the academic elite of medicine, who I would think should be paid and encouraged to be more open-minded than the rest of us.

Smart people were talking and writing about low-glycemic-index diets for a long time, as I cited in the text, doctors educated at top U.S. medical schools. Why weren't opposing theories given a fair shot at the height of the gung-ho, all-fat-is-bad days?

Isn't science's job to consider all the possibilities, test for them in controlled experiments, throw out ideas proved wrong, refine ideas proved right, do more experimenting, until gradually, inexorably we approach some great universal truth?

Well…I used to think so.

Yet my own experience has not always shown science to work that way.

Several times in my career I have encountered instances—the low-fat/low-carb question being one—where it seems to me experts wear bizarre blinders about even contemplating dogma-threatening new ideas.

And, stunningly, I stumbled upon an explanation—or, at least, objective confirmation of my observations—during my writing of this book. Thomas S. Kuhn (1922–1996), a Harvard-trained physicist turned historian and philosopher of science, published a landmark book in 1962 titled, *The Structure of Scientific Revolutions*. In this book, he tossed out that notion I had, most of us have: that romantic view of science as—quoting Jeffery Kasser of North Carolina State University— "straightforwardly cumulative, progressive, or truth-tracking."

This traditional, romanticized image of science, according to philosopher Kasser, included an "openness to criticism," and almost obsession with *disproving* itself—after all, the more times you fail to disprove something the more strongly can be its claim of truthfulness—that Kuhn felt did not exist in real-world science.

Normal science, in Kuhn's view, is governed instead by *paradigms*. A paradigm is an object of consensus not open to criticism. The paradigm is assumed to be correct. It is dogma. It determines the puzzles to be solved, which involve fitting nature into the paradigm, and defines the expected results, and the standards for evaluating those results. Science doesn't seek truth, it seeks to prove the paradigm.

Dietary fat is unhealthy and the main promoter of obesity was the paradigm governing academic medicine's evaluation of low-fat versus low-carb dieting (i.e., the glycemic-index question) twenty years ago, and few mainstream researchers were motivated, encouraged, or funded to do research other than for the purpose of proving that proposition.

Another example of a paradigm—a shaky paradigm to my thinking—in my sub-specialized area of medicine involves defining a person's thyroid-function almost solely in terms of blood thyroid-stimulating hormone (TSH) testing. Without going into details (I talk a lot about this in my book *The Thyroid Paradox*), the paradigm is that a TSH level virtually always accurately assesses thyroid function, both in clinical practice and in research. If thyroid levels are low, for example, the TSH test almost always will read high, or so goes the dogma. Much of the time, yes, but I don't think any test is as reliable as this one is usually given credit for. Now, in clinical practice, it is possible for a good thyroidologist to thoroughly evaluate the patient, confirm that the evident signs and symptoms agree with the TSH level, and make an appropriate decision. I'm not saying all doctors taking care of thyroid patients do that—that is, read between the lines of a "normal" TSH and decide the patient has low thyroid function (hypothyroidism) anyway—but it is possible for them to do so. There is a bigger problem, to my thinking, with scientific papers—looking at questions like, *Does environmental pollutant X kill thyroid function?*—basing their conclusions largely, if not exclusively on TSH testing. I look at papers of that ilk with a very big grain of salt, in case the paradigm is wrong.

One more case in point:

When I was in the Air Force, many veterans of 1991's Persian Gulf War were presenting with unexplained illnesses, that became known as "Gulf War Syndrome" (GWS). An edict came down from the Pentagon that we were to drop everything and evaluate large numbers of these veterans to determine if there was a basis for their complaints. In effect: was GWS real? Rather than approach the assignment with an open, objective mind, however, like I thought we should, putting on our scientific investigator hats, it was my disturbed observation that most of us were just out to prove the *paradigm* that GWS didn't exist. I'm not saying these veterans didn't get the evaluation they were supposed to—they did—but the attitude with which I saw the task approached, seemed more in accordance with Kuhn's notions of real-world science, then one would like to see.

In the Kuhn view, a *scientific crisis* occurs when the paradigm loses its grip, when the puzzles resist solution (failure of low-fat dieting to quell the epidemic of obesity??), and confidence in the paradigm is lost. It is during a crisis that the paradigm is questioned, tested, and perhaps rejected. When a new paradigm takes over, Kuhn calls this a *scientific revolution.* Older scientists resist; they have their careers invested, after all, in the old paradigm. Younger ones make the switch more readily, the old paradigm slowly dying off, literally, as its proponents do.

My discovery of Kuhn was an epiphany, explaining and confirming what was seeming to me blatant bias driving what should be open-minded scientific inquiry. Now, if that's the way the world works, so be it. The world is what it is, and it is certainly not perfect. It concerns me greatly though if a product of this biased system—some medical association's clinical-practice guidelines for management of disease Q, for example—is used by evidence-based medicine, and health insurers, insurers wielding in one instance the full weight and power of the federal government, to decide how doctors should treat disease Q and what tests and drugs and surgeries might be paid for.

And I have other concerns—beyond Kuhnian bias—about the role of the randomized, prospective, controlled clinical trial, and other study models, as the end-all-be-all of medical decision making, and medical knowledge in general. They are useful to be sure, even vital—but they are not *everything*, as I fear is the current paradigm.

For example, as good and as careful as researchers are, they can't mimic the complex conditions of the real world that real patients are immersed in. For valid reasons, studies are crafted to focus on one, or a limited number of parameters. Say we want to know if Drug K or Industrial Waste Product Triple-Z causes pancreatic cancer. Researchers will assemble two groups of subjects that are as much alike as they can manage, except that one group is exposed to Drug K or Product Triple-Z, and the other group isn't, then they sit back and count the number of pancreatic cancers showing up in each group. Now, I want to know the results of that trial, and I'll take it into account. However, I have patients taking twenty different drugs. I might be prescribing four diabetes drugs to an individual, and his cardiologist might be prescribing four heart drugs and we haven't even discussed his neurologist, his podiatrist, his internist. Say, Drug K is shown in our hypothetical study to not increase the risk of pancreatic cancer. Okay, and say I add it to the twenty drugs my patient is already taking, confident it doesn't cause pancreatic cancer.

How do I know there aren't three other drugs on his list, now interacting with Drug K, and that four-drug cocktail isn't a potent promoter of pancreatic cancer? It doesn't have to be other drugs. Maybe he is exposed to Industrial Waste Product Triple-Z. And while neither Product Triple-Z nor Drug K cause pancreatic cancer by themselves, maybe the combination does 99 percent of the time. Or maybe he has an obscure cancer-promoting gene that lies dormant until it is activated by Drug K.

My point is, the randomized controlled trial's look at one or very few variables against a background of supposed uniformity is both a great strength and great weakness, for human populations are anything but uniform. We have to do medical research and we should pay attention to it, but we cannot assume those results give us anywhere close to a full understanding of real-world human pathophysiology, and yet we keep blundering along as if they do. Now, there comes a time when a medical decision needs to be made, whether or not we feel we have all the facts to make the best decision. We do as well as we can in that situation. Worst case scenario: say it was the wrong decision and the patient suffers for it. That's tragic, but at the end of the day, it's one doctor and one patient. Where I have a problem is when public policies get formulated and implemented based on this intrinsically flawed research, policies that affect millions of lives. Like the disastrous original Food Guide Pyramid.

I might go so far as to say that government should stay out of giving or mandating medical advice. Or perhaps it should limit itself to banning or regulating the "proven harmful," and refrain from promoting the "supposed beneficial." I say this because it is a principle of logic that you can't prove a negative. Meaning: I can never prove something doesn't ever do harm. I can prove something does do harm, though, by pointing to a single case of harm. And if there are enough clear cases of harm, and the harm is great enough, then and only then, I would argue, should government interfere.

If you've stuck with me this far, now I'm really going to dive into some biostatistical esoterica. Hang on as I take a swipe at the greatest sacred cow in all of science and statistical analysis.

The greatest, most entrenched paradigm of all!

The lowly p-value.

"P" standing for *probability*.

When data from any experiment is analyzed, it must be determined whether the results from one group differ from another group—supporting the hypothesis that Group A is different from Group B for some reason—and if they are different, is that difference *statistically significant?*

The question, about statistical significance, that in reality gets asked is:

What is the probability that the *null hypothesis*—the hypothesis that Groups A and B are *not* different—is true in spite of the data?

Under the conditions of the experiment, what are the chances the results could have come from random chance, rather than as a consequence of a true difference between the groups? And if that probability is sufficiently small (a low p-value), the results are said to be statistically significant and the experiment is said to show the groups are different.

If, however, the probability that the null hypothesis is true is large (a high p-value), then the data are said to have not achieved significance, and the groups are said to be no different. In which case, that particular experiment goes down in the annals of science as failing to show a difference between Groups A and B. If the question is an important one, more than one experiment will be done, and if all the studies agree there is a difference, or there isn't a difference, then consensus is reached and, assuming we all agree that enough of the work was conducted properly, everybody is happy with whatever the answer is.

If some experiments draw one conclusion, though, and others draw a different one, that's when things get confusing. That's when we get a news item one week saying Vitamin Triple-X is good for us, and one next week saying it causes heart attacks.

That's when we need to do bigger better studies.

This is all good and useful. We obviously need some method we all can agree upon to look at sets of data and decide if they tell us anything. My gripe is with where the line is drawn, between statistical significance, and nonsignificance.

It's an important question because in medicine today, if a certain test, or certain treatment is studied and the data as to their usefulness is deemed not significant, then that test or treatment has a good chance of being thrown away, or at least not supported under evidence-based medicine, meaning insurance might not pay for it.

A p-value of 5 percent is that cutoff virtually universally in all scientific research.

If p is less than 5 percent, a study's results are said to be statistically significant, and we pay attention to whatever a cursory exam of the data already told us. We are saying there is a less than 5 percent chance the null hypothesis could be true given the data. If p is greater or equal to 5%, then the results are deemed not significant, no matter what an eyeballing of the data might suggest. In other words, if Drug Alpha cures people 75% of the time, but the p-value is 10 percent (a 10 percent chance that the null hypothesis—that Drug Alpha is worthless—is true despite the attractive data) then Drug Alpha is going to be discredited or at least have to wait for another experiment.

Why 5 percent?

Why is 5 percent the magic p-value?

Surely there is some sound statistical reasoning, right?

No… not so much…

It was an arbitrary threshold set by one man, Cambridge geneticist and statistician R.A. Fisher, in 1926, in a paper published in the *Journal of the Ministry of Agriculture of Great Britain*. In that paper he discusses the pros and cons of various p cutoffs, and states, "Personally, the writer prefers...the 5 per cent point."

Now, I'm not arguing against a 5 percent p-value threshold. It's a perfectly reasonable number, if we have to have just one number. What I am arguing against, am flabbergasted by, is that under the potential tyranny of evidence-based medicine, all medical decision making would, in theory, be subjected to a p-value analysis, and any and all major patient-care interventions would be accepted or rejected on the basis of whether the p was greater or less than 5 percent, a number that sounded good to one man 86 years ago.

What's wrong with 4.5 percent, or 3 percent, or 6.35 percent?

Especially in this age of highly accurate, push-of-a-button, computer computations, in which multi-page tables in the backs of statistics textbooks are obsolete, any reasonable figure could be chosen. Don't tell me a treatment rejected because of a p equal to 6.0002 percent is really all that less likely to be helpful to some people than a treatment that lucked out with a p of 4.9997%.

I think the whole notion of p-values should be revamped.

My proposal, if anybody cares: ignore all results failing to reach a significance indicated by a p of, say, 10 percent, but for each study—ahead of time, *a priori*, that's extremely important to assuring integrity—the investigators conducting the research will establish the p-value threshold of significance for that particular study, a value anywhere between 9.9999% and, say, 1.0000%, or possibly less. The p-value would no longer be arbitrary, because its selection would be based upon the relative cost of a wrong conclusion, a risk-benefit analysis, which is already part and parcel of good medicine.

If we are investigating the efficacy of Drug Y against Disease Q, we might set a high p-value threshold of, say, 9 percent if Drug Y is very safe and Disease Q is a nonfatal nuisance, on the order of the common cold.

Whereas if Drug Y has a dangerous collection of side effects and Disease Q is almost always fatal, you wouldn't want to deem Drug Y to be an acceptable treatment unless you were pretty darned sure it worked. An appropriate significance threshold in that situation might be less than 1 percent, or perhaps, less than 0.1 percent. Any number in between the defined extremes might be chosen depending on the exact combination of risks and benefits intrinsic to the situation being studied.

Such a system would be chaos deployed throughout the scientific community, across all fields. I do think, however, such a system—

admittedly and intentionally complex—should be considered for the biomedical, or at least medical sciences. Medicine is complex and diverse, and the same set of standards cannot be applied to all situations. One important example of complexity in medicine which does not exist in, say, astrophysics, is that there can be important, even fatal costs to both overcaution and overboldness. As many people could, hypothetically, die from the rejection of an effective treatment, as could from acceptance of a dangerous or ineffective one.

ABOUT THE AUTHOR

James K. Rone, MD, is a writer and board-certified endocrinologist in Murfreesboro, Tennessee where he has been in private practice since 1998. Before that he was a U.S. Air Force physician for eleven years. Dr. Rone is a Fellow of the American College of Physicians and the American College of Endocrinology; he holds memberships in numerous professional organizations, including the American and European Thyroid Associations, the American Diabetes Association, The Endocrine Society, and The Obesity Society. Besides over a quarter century of clinical experience, Dr. Rone is a diabetes and thyroid patient himself. He lives with his wife, Susan, three horses, two cats, and a dog named Emma, on their farm outside Nashville.